# Social Work Doctoral Education

T0227968

The rapid expansion of doctoral education in social work is changing academia and expanding the expectations of education for professional practice. This volume focuses on the early development, gradual evolution and present status of social work doctoral education. Relevant for social work students and educators globally, it represents an authoritative statement authored by widely recognized educators who are on the cutting edge of doctoral education.

Documenting the current state of the art, this comprehensive book demonstrates the rapidly growing importance of doctoral-level education in the social work profession. The authors look closely at current trends and address the emerging pedagogical issues that will likely frame the future.

This book was originally published as a special issue of the *Journal of Teaching in Social Work*.

**Paul A. Kurzman, Ph.D., ACSW** holds a dual appointment as a Professor of Social Work at the Silberman School at Hunter College, NY, USA, and as a Professor of Social Welfare at the Graduate School and University Center of the City University of New York, NY, USA, where he teaches policy and practice in the MSW and Ph.D. programs. He also is the Editor in Chief of the *Journal of Teaching in Social Work* and a member of the Editorial Board of the *Journal of Workplace Behavioral Health*. Dr. Kurzman served for a record 26 years on the New York State Social Work Licensing Board, chaired the board of the first *Register of Clinical Social Workers*, was elected the President of the Faculty of Hunter College, and was appointed Acting Dean of the School of Social Work. Professor Kurzman has held major leadership positions in the National Association of Social Workers, locally and nationally, including as President of the New York City Chapter, from which he recently received their Lifetime Achievement Award. He is an author or editor of nine prior books, including *Union Contributions to Labor Welfare Policy and Practice* (with R.P. Maiden); *Work and the Workplace: A Resource for Innovative Policy and Practice* (with S. Akabas); *Labor and Industrial Settings: Sites for Social Work Practice* (with S. Akabas and N. Kolben); *Psychosocial and Policy Issues in the World of Work, Work, Workers and Work Organizations: A View from Social Work* (with S. Akabas); *Harry Hopkins and the New Deal*; *Work and Well-being: The Occupational Social Work Advantage* (with S. Akabas); *Distance Learning and Online Education in Social Work* (with R.P. Maiden); and *The Mississippi Experience: Strategies for Welfare Rights Action*. Dr. Kurzman holds a BA from Princeton University, an MSW from Columbia University and a Ph.D. from New York University. He can be reached at pkurzman@hunter.cuny.edu.

# Social Work Doctoral Education

Past, present and future

*Edited by*
**Paul A. Kurzman**

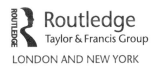

Routledge
Taylor & Francis Group

LONDON AND NEW YORK

First published 2016
by Routledge
2 Park Square, Milton Park, Abingdon, Oxon, OX14 4RN, UK

and by Routledge
711 Third Avenue, New York, NY 10017, USA

First issued in paperback 2017

*Routledge is an imprint of the Taylor & Francis Group, an informa business*

© 2016 Taylor & Francis

All rights reserved. No part of this book may be reprinted or reproduced or utilised in any form or by any electronic, mechanical, or other means, now known or hereafter invented, including photocopying and recording, or in any information storage or retrieval system, without permission in writing from the publishers.

*Trademark notice*: Product or corporate names may be trademarks or registered trademarks, and are used only for identification and explanation without intent to infringe.

*British Library Cataloguing in Publication Data*
A catalogue record for this book is available from the British Library

ISBN 13: 978-1-138-29504-9 (pbk)
ISBN 13: 978-1-138-95322-2 (hbk)

Typeset in Garamond
by diacriTech, Chennai

**Publisher's Note**
The publisher accepts responsibility for any inconsistencies that may have arisen during the conversion of this book from journal articles to book chapters, namely the possible inclusion of journal terminology.

**Disclaimer**
Every effort has been made to contact copyright holders for their permission to reprint material in this book. The publishers would be grateful to hear from any copyright holder who is not here acknowledged and will undertake to rectify any errors or omissions in future editions of this book.

# Contents

# CONTENTS

# Citation Information

The chapters in this book were originally published in the *Journal of Teaching in Social Work*, volume 35, issues 1–2 (Jan–June 2015). When citing this material, please use the original page numbering for each article, as follows:

**Chapter 13**

*Writing for Publication: Assessment of a Course for Social Work Doctoral Students*
Deena Mandell, Hend Shalan, Carol Stalker, and Lea Caragata
*Journal of Teaching in Social Work*, volume 35, issues 1–2 (Jan–June 2015)
pp. 197–212

**Chapter 14**

*Building Scholarly Writers: Student Perspectives on Peer Review in a Doctoral Writing Seminar*
Margaret Ellen Adamek
*Journal of Teaching in Social Work*, volume 35, issues 1–2 (Jan–June 2015)
pp. 213–225

**Chapter 15: Conclusion**

*Doctoral Education in Social Work: An Essay Review*
Bruce A. Thyer
*Journal of Teaching in Social Work*, volume 35, issues 1–2 (Jan–June 2015)
pp. 226–229

For any permissions-related enquiries please visit
http://www.tandfonline.com/page/help/permissions

# Notes on Contributors

**Margaret Ellen Adamek, Ph.D.** is a Professor and Director of the Ph.D. Program in Social Work at Indiana University in Indianapolis, IN, USA, and can be reached at madamek@iupui.edu.

**Bree Akesson, Ph.D.** is an Assistant Professor on the Faculty of Social Work at Wilfred Laurier University, Waterloo, Canada, and can be reached at bakesson@wlu.ca.

**Laura Berenson, Ph.D., LCSW** is a Lecturer at the Silberman School of Social Work at Hunter College, City University of New York, NY, USA, and can be reached at laberenson@gmail.com.

**Roni Berger, Ph.D.** is a Professor in the School of Social Work at Adelphi University, NY, USA, and can be reached at berger@adelphi.edu.

**Joan Berzoff, Ed.D.** is a Professor in the School for Social Work at Smith College, Northampton, Massachusetts, USA, and can be reached at Jberzoff@smith.edu.

**Anne Blumenthal, MSW** is a Ph.D. candidate in the School of Social Work at the University of Michigan, Ann Arbor, MI, USA, and can be reached at Anneblue@umich.edu.

**Lea Caragata, Ph.D.** is a Professor and Associate Dean for the Ph.D. Program at the Faculty of Social Work of Wilfrid Laurier University, Waterloo, Canada, and can be reached at lcaragata@wlu.ca.

**Mollie Lazar Charter, MSW** is a Doctoral candidate at the School of Social Work at the University of Connecticut, Mansfield, CT, USA, and can be reached at mollie.charter@uconn.edu.

**James P. Coyle, Ph.D., RSW** is an Associate Professor in the School of Social Work at the University of Windsor, Canada, and can be reached at jcoyle@windsor.ca.

**Mery Diaz, DSW, LCSW** is an Assistant Professor in the Health and Human Services Department at New York City College of Technology, NY, USA, and can be reached at mdiaz@citytech.cuny.edu.

**Matthew Ditty, DSW, LCSW** is a part-time Lecturer at the School of Social Policy and Practice of the University of Pennsylvania, Philadelphia, PA, USA, and can be reached at mdit@sp2.upenn.edu.

**Andrea Doyle, Ph.D., LCSW** is an Assistant Professor at the School of Social Policy and Practice of the University of Pennsylvania, Philadelphia, PA, USA, and can be reached at doylea@sp2.upenn.edu

**James Drisko, Ph.D., LICSW** is a Professor in the School for Social Work at Smith College, Northampton, MA, USA, and can be reached at jdrisko@smith.edu.

**Harriet Goodman, DSW, LMSW** is an Associate Professor at the Silberman School of Social Work at Hunter College, and Executive Officer of the Ph.D. Program in Social Welfare at the Graduate Center of the City University of New York, NY, USA, and can be reached at hgoodman@hunter.cuny.edu.

**Cynthia L. Grant, Ph.D., LCSW** is the Quality Improvement Clinical Manager at Arapahoe/Douglas Mental Health Network in Englewood, CO, USA, and Lecturer at the School of Education and Human Development at the University of Colorado in Denver, CO, USA. She can be reached at grant.lcsw@gmail.com.

**Robin M. Hartinger-Saunders, Ph.D., LMSW** is an Assistant Professor at the School of Social Work at Georgia State University, Atlanta, GA, USA, and can be reached at rsaunders@gsu.edu.

**Lina Hartocollis, Ph.D., LCSW** is an Adjunct Assistant Professor and Director of the Clinical DSW Program at the School of Social Policy and Practice of the University of Pennsylvania, Philadelphia, PA, USA, and can be reached at lhartoco@sp2.upenn.edu.

**Christie Hunnicutt, LCSW** is a Ph.D. candidate in the School for Social Work at Smith College, Northampton, MA, USA, and can be reached at chunnicutt@smith.edu.

**Kelly F. Jackson, Ph.D.** is an Associate Professor in the School of Social Work at Arizona State University, Tempe, AZ, USA, and can be reached at kelly.f.jackson@asu.edu.

**Susan Patricia Kemp, Ph.D.** is the Charles O. Cressey Associate Professor at the School of Social Work at the University of Washington, Seattle, WA, USA, and can be reached at spk@uw.edu.

**Paul A. Kurzman, Ph.D., ACSW** is a Professor at the Silberman School of Social Work at Hunter College, and a Professor of Social Welfare at the Graduate Center of the City University of New York, NY, USA, and can be reached at pkurzman@hunter.cuny.edu.

**Lucyna Lach, Ph.D.** is an Associate Professor at the School of Social Work at McGill University, Montreal, Canada, and can be reached at lucy.lach@mcgill.ca.

**Elaine M. Maccio, Ph.D., LCSW** is an Associate Professor at the School of Social Work of Louisiana State University, Baton Rouge, LA, USA, and can be reached at emaccio@lsu.edu.

**Deena Mandell, Ph.D.** is an Associate Professor of the Faculty of Social Work at Wilfrid Laurier University, Waterloo, Canada, and can be reached at dmandell@wlu.ca.

**Cristina Mogro-Wilson, Ph.D.** is an Associate Professor at the School of Social Work of the University of Connecticut, Mansfield, CT, USA, and can be reached at cristina.wilson@uconn.edu.

**Paula S. Nurius, Ph.D.** is a Professor and Grace Beals-Ferguson Scholar at the School of Social Work at Washington University, St Louis, MO, USA, and can be reached at nurius@u.washington.edu.

**Michael G. Reeves, MSW**, is a Doctoral candidate at the School of Social Work of the University of Connecticut, Mansfield, CT, USA, and can be reached at michael.reeves@uconn.edu.

**Christine M. Rine, Ph.D., LMSW** is an Assistant Professor in the Department of Social Work of Edinboro University of Pennsylvania, PA, USA, and can be reached at crine@edinboro.edu.

**Elaine S. Rinfrette, Ph.D., LCSW** is an Assistant Professor in the Department of Social Work of Edinboro University of Pennsylvania, PA, USA, and can be reached at erinfrette@edinboro.edu.

**David W. Rothwell, Ph.D.** is an Assistant Professor and Director of the Ph.D. Program at the School of Social Work at McGill University, Montreal, Canada, and can be reached at rothwell@mcgill.ca.

**Hend Shalan, M.Ed.** is a Ph.D. candidate in social work at Wilfrid Laurier University, Waterloo, Canada, and can be reached at shal8310@mylaurier.ca.

**Lawrence Shulman, Ed.D.** is a Professor and Dean Emeritus at the University at Buffalo of the State University of New York, NY, USA, and can be reached at shulman@buffalo.edu.

**Phyllis Solomon, Ph.D.** is a Professor at the School of Social Policy and Practice of the University of Pennsylvania, Philadelphia, PA, USA, and can be reached at solomonp@sp2.upenn.edu.

**Carol Stalker, Ph.D**, is a Professor on the Faculty of Social Work at Wilfrid Laurier University, Waterloo, Canada, and can be reached at cstalker@wlu.ca.

**Bruce A. Thyer, Ph.D., LCSW** is a Professor in the College of Social Work at Florida State University, Tallahassee, FL, USA, and can be reached at bthyer@fsu.edu.

**Daniel R. Tomal, Ph.D.** is a Distinguished Professor of Leadership in the College of Graduate and Innovative Programs at Concordia University of Chicago, IL, USA, and can be reached at daniel.tomal@chuchicago.edu.

# Acknowledgements

When we issued a Call for Papers for a book on *Social Work Doctoral Education* we had not imagined the response it would receive. While we knew this to be a cutting-edge issue, which prompted our interest in taking the initiative, the sheer number of excellent manuscripts we received, for the journal's special issue and hence the book, certainly did surprise us! Our belief that the time had come for a new and authoritative text on the subject had been validated, and we hope the peer-reviewed selection of these 15 superb chapters confirms that conviction to the reader. Representing the ideas of 36 contributing authors, the chapters herein present new information, novel experimentation, fresh conceptualization and creative templates for what surely represents an important thrust for professional social work education in the future.

As Editor, I am very grateful for the can-do spirit and steady support of Helen Stuhr-Rommereim, Managing Editor for Behavioral Science and Social Care, Emily Ross, Editor of Routledge Special Issues as Books, Nicholas Barclay, Editorial Assistant, and Elizabeth T. Kerr, Production Editor at the Taylor & Francis Group. Their patience and flexibility made a difference. And it is clear that this book would not have been possible without the quiet, steady and focused support of Ruth Flaherty, the Assistant Editor of the *Journal of Teaching in Social Work*, who carried out so many of the tasks of assignment and production with an always skillful and steady hand.

And to the contributors, whose insights and innovations are so articulately expressed here, we give thanks and tribute for their remarkable creativity and their insightful innovations. In this book, each of them individually, and all of them collectively, have made an indelible professional contribution to the future of doctoral social work education

Paul A. Kurzman
August 2015

# The Evolution of Doctoral Social Work Education

PAUL A. KURZMAN

*Silberman School of Social Work, Hunter College, The City University of New York, New York, New York, USA*

*Doctoral education in social work is evolving as a major enterprise in American higher education, with more than 80 programs now in place. Committed to providing stewards of the profession, these PhD and DSW programs also are a major impetus for research and are the primary faculty pipeline for the 735 CSWE-accredited professional social work education programs in the country. Past achievements, current challenges, and present trends are discussed here, along with the principal issues facing doctoral programs in the decade ahead.*

## INTRODUCTION

Over the past 95 years, doctoral social work education has grown from infancy to adulthood. Beginning with programs at Bryn Mawr College and the University of Chicago in 1920, the enterprise grew slowly at the beginning, with merely eight programs in place 30 years later. Today, in 2015, there are more than 2,500 students enrolled in more than 80 recognized programs in the United States and Canada, with many more present abroad and emerging in developing nations across the globe (Council on Social Work Education [CSWE], 2013; Group for the Advancement of Doctoral Education in Social Work [GADE], 2015; Lubben, 2008). The Great Depression surely slowed the growth of programs during the 1930s, along with World War

1

II and the economic recovery of the 1940s, as well as the unanticipated economic impact of the Korean Conflict in the early 1950s. However, a sudden surge in doctoral programs took place in the 1960s and 1970s with the emergence of President Kennedy's and President Johnson's innovative social programs. Indeed, 20 new social work doctoral programs were initiated between 1965 and 1975 (Van Scoy, 1978).

The social work versus social welfare identity crisis (of which some authors write) was evident at the schools that launched the early doctoral courses of study. None of the initial doctoral programs was under the auspices of what was termed a "school of social work" or a "school of social welfare"—the usual dyad. Early doctoral program sponsors were the Bryn Mawr Graduate School of Social Work and Social Research [1920] and the University of Chicago School of Social Service Administration [1920]—both awarding the PhD—and the Catholic University School of Social Service [1947] and the University of Pennsylvania School of Social Policy and Practice [1948]—granting the Doctor of Social Work (DSW) degree. It was not until 50 years later that a greater uniformity of nomenclature emerged and that some clarification was achieved with respect to the differences and similarities of the two degrees granted. In fact, some would say that such clarity is still in the eyes of the beholder.

Although the DSW degree was most common upon the expansion of programs in the late 1960s through the 1970s, pressure toward an emphasis on scholarship and research gradually became a driving force toward the emerging dominance of PhD degree programs. New social work doctoral programs were virtually universal in offering the PhD from this time forward, and most existing DSW programs converted to awarding the PhD, making very modest changes in their requirements or their curricula in the process (Anastas & Kuerbis, 2009). By the 1990s, the award of the DSW degree had all but vanished; however, it reemerged during the next two decades as a complement to the now standard and prevalent social work PhD (Anastas, 2012). Indeed, universities that offer the DSW degree today (such as Tennessee, NYU, Rutgers, and Pennsylvania) do so not *instead of* by rather *in addition to* the PhD.

Some authors feel that the revival of the DSW degree is a legitimate (in fact essential) response to the need both for practitioners who can conduct practice-based research and for senior clinicians who can take on leadership positions in public and nonprofit agency settings, where the doctoral degree increasingly has become an expectation. As one scholar observed,

> A Doctoral Program in Social Work practice (DSW) is a timely development in social work education. . . . Throughout the world and in the United States, various professions and practical disciplines have moved into developing doctoral level education that is not geared for research

but to produce highly qualified practitioners who are capable of engaging in practice-related research. (Cnaan, as cited in Anastas, 2012, p. 32)

Others see the emerging focus on the DSW degree alternative as a way of responding to the shortage of young faculty (with social work doctorates) to fill the growing need of the current 735 CSWE-accredited social work programs in the United States (CSWE, 2015). However, some (Raymond & Valentine, 2001) perceive the promotion of the professional DSW primarily as a "prestige quest" of the profession.

Award of the professional doctorate of course has a long and revered history, for such a degree has generally been the tradition in America and abroad for our most august professions, such as medicine (MD), dentistry (DDS), and more recently the law (JD). Few would question the prestige and authority of these professions and of the holders of their *practice* doctorates, so those who possess the DSW degree could be said to travel in good company.

One must also acknowledge the quiet trend over the past 20 years toward the "upgrading" of professional degrees among a great many of our sister health and mental health professions. Although the National Association of Social Workers (NASW) and CSWE still consider the MSW to be the "terminal professional degree", and none of the 50 states currently mandates a doctoral degree for licensure to practice, there is pressure upon the organizational and educational gatekeepers of the social work profession to consider the long-range implications of choosing not to follow the present trend of its peer professions (NASW, 2013). Recently, most of the allied professions, with whom we work and compete, have made a professional doctorate the entry-level degree for practice of their profession, and they have successfully promoted this expectation to their state licensing boards and national accrediting organizations. Although some distinguished social work educators express concern about the general movement in this direction (Khinduka, 2002; Reisch, 2002), the trend is difficult to deny. By way of example, audiologists must now have an AudD, nutritionists a DSN, physical therapists a DPT, psychologists a PhD or PsyD, and occupational therapists an OTD. All, like the DSW, are professional degrees, patterned after the one that is held by physicians (MD), which they likely wish to emulate. Many will argue: Where will this explicit trend leave social work if it chooses not to promote the doctorate as an option—perhaps even the expectation—for social work licensure? Because recent data show that in the past 20 years there has been a significant increase in the proportion of social work doctoral programs located in what the well-respected Carnegie Foundation Classification System would term "non-research focused universities," the adoption of a DSW degree option (with less focus on research) may prove to be a good fit, if sought by our profession (Anastas, 2006; Lubben, 2008).

## PREPARING GRADUATES TO TEACH

It is universally acknowledged that a principal role of doctoral social work education is to prepare graduates for teaching in the current 233 MSW and 502 BSW CSWE-accredited programs in the United States and the many recognized social work programs abroad. The institutional needs of these programs have grown in recent years; CSWE data show that there were 11,425 social work faculty (full time + part time) in 2013, up from 9,825 merely 2 years prior (CSWE, 2015, p. 19). Furthermore, a great number of these faculty members are now approaching retirement age. Simply stated, Zastrow and Bremner (2004) underscore the reality that there now is a severe shortage of qualified candidates for available junior faculty positions, in both graduate and undergraduate programs, and that this fact is likely to persist (indeed grow) over the next few decades. The shortfall is particularly acute, they noted, in the production of social work doctoral graduates who have an MSW and who therefore are eligible to teach practice.

GADE is the principal external organization with the goal of promoting quality in doctoral social work education. Without a central office or full-time staff, GADE functions effectively yet informally to coordinate and represent most of the doctoral programs in the United States and Canada. It operates a website and a listserv and holds an annual meeting, which most doctoral program chairpersons attend. GADE is not an accrediting association, like CSWE, but does promulgate guidelines and standards to promote excellence in both PhD and DSW degree education (Lubben, 2008). In a recent report (GADE, 2013, p. 3), their Task Force on Quality Guidelines noted that "PhD programs of all types have long been criticized for failing to adequately prepare students to teach" and recommended that all social work PhD students have "independently taught at least one course at the BSW and/or MSW level as the instructor of record" (p. 6) prior to graduation, a position supported by a number of scholars (Anastas, 2010; Knight & Lagana, 1999; Valentine et al., 1998).

Equally important, it would appear that fewer and fewer doctoral students are choosing to enter academia upon graduation. Findings from Jeane Anastas's seminal 2007 survey showed then that approximately 50% to 60% of social work doctoral graduates moved into faculty positions (Anastas, 2012, p. 172), whereas CSWE 2012–2013 statistics (CSWE, 2013, p. 40) indicate that, merely 5 years later, only 35.2% of such graduates had moved into a tenure line faculty position in an accredited program.

In response to the growing need for doctoral graduates to choose academia as a career, particularly as faculty who will be qualified to teach practice, several new programs have emerged. Saint Catherine University and the University of Saint Thomas in Minnesota recently have jointly initiated a new DSW program focused "on preparing social work faculty specifically for university level teaching and leadership in higher education" (University of

St. Thomas, n.d.). Courses on curriculum development and educational pedagogy (along with classroom and field teaching) are required, and every candidate must pursue a supervised teaching practicum as well. Equally important, applicants must have an MSW degree and at least 2 years' postmaster's social work practice experience. (This experience requirement is an effective response to Proctor's, 1996, and Munson's, 1996, classic debate on this subject.) Further, Rutgers University (n.d.) recently launched a new DSW degree option (to complement its ongoing research-centered PhD program) which is designed to meet the need for advanced clinical social work practitioners and educators (Royeen & Lavin, 2007). In addition, the University of Southern California, the largest school of social work in the nation and a nationally ranked leader, has started a new DSW program in the fall of 2015 with a track specifically focused on "advanced evidence-based clinical practice," which will be offered via a hybrid online and onsite model of instruction (Flynn, Maiden, Smith, Wiley, & Wood, 2013, p. 355). Moreover, two independent social work PhD programs (which are not members of GADE and do not offer the MSW degree) concentrate solely on the preparation of advanced social work clinicians, primarily for teaching in academia and for leadership positions in clinical settings: The California Institute for Clinical Social Work (also known as the Sanville Institute), and The Institute for Clinical Social Work in Illinois. Finally, two for-profit institutions, Capella University and Walden University, are both offering DSW degree programs, with a concentration on clinical practice, leadership, and teaching. Given these several initiatives, perhaps preparation of an increasing number of doctoral graduates (and therefore potential new faculty) with *clinical practice* experience will mean that this particular practice-focused cohort will no longer be what Johnson and Munch (2010) termed the "dinosaurs" among doctoral social work faculty.

## THE ROLE OF THE DSW DEGREE

As we have noted, reappearance of the DSW degree in recent years has been a significant factor in the evolution and maturation of doctoral social work education. A GADE task force, chaired by Richard Edwards, past president of NASW and then dean of the Rutgers University School of Social Work, came forward with an influential report, "The Doctorate in Social Work (DSW) Degree: Emergence of a New Practice Doctorate" (GADE, 2011). Two years later, the NASW Social Work Policy Institute in Washington, DC convened an invitational symposium titled "Advanced Practice Doctorates: What Do They Mean for Social Work Practice, Research and Education?" A strong case was made at the symposium, by a dean of one of the graduate schools currently offering the degree, that DSW programs could advance not only practice knowledge and skills but practice-related research as well. Moreover, from a practical standpoint, it was pointed out that the DSW degree might effectively enhance social work's marketability, as a profession, as its graduates compete with those of sister professions, especially psychology where the doctorate (PhD, PsyD) has become the norm (Pace, 2013, p. 4).

Whereas CSWE statistics show that 94.4% of social work doctoral degrees awarded during the academic year 2012–2013 were PhDs (CSWE, 2013, p. 38), DSW degrees are a small but growing subset that warrants attention and recognition. Upon completion of her 2007 landmark study of the doctorate, Anastas (2012) noted that

> social work is experiencing a "crisis" in doctoral education [that] has most often been described as a shortage of applicants to and graduates from doctoral programs in schools of social work despite a steady increase in the number of doctoral programs housed in schools of social work. (p. 3)

Many propose that the DSW—to complement and to supplement the PhD— could be part of the solution (O'Neill, 2000; Orme, 2003; Robb, 2005). Conceptualized by the 2011 GADE task force, previously noted, the DSW would be conceived and redesigned as an Advanced Practice Doctorate, analogous to the PsyD in psychology. Indeed, the Task Force Report (GADE, 2011) noted that

> academic institutions have indicated a growing need for faculty holding a terminal [doctoral] degree in the profession who trained as advanced practitioners and come into academe with a strong practice background. This [DSW] degree would further the recruitment efforts for practitioner scholars on faculties nationally and internationally. (p. 8)

Although most DSW graduates may choose to pursue leadership roles as advanced practitioners, a great many likely would select a career in academia—teaching social work practice, developing new instructional modalities for incorporation into their school's human behavior and the social environment and practice curricula, and collaborating with research colleagues on securing grants for innovative outreach to underserved client populations. In this manner, DSW graduates may well serve plural needs, including greater access to government agency leadership positions, advancing the current knowledge base for professional practice, and meeting present and prospective needs of the academy.

## THE FUNCTION OF ONLINE PROGRAMS

One response to the shortage of doctoral social work graduates has been the offering of more and more doctoral courses via distance education. Although many current PhD programs are providing an option for students to take a portion of their courses online, leadership in this direction would appear to be coming more from the emerging DSW programs. The DSW options being offered by the University of Tennessee, Aurora University, and Rutgers University, for example, provide a great deal of course instruction through a variety of distance learning arrangements; and the newest DSW program, jointly sponsored by Saint Catherine University and the University of Saint Thomas (which have hosted collaborative CSWE-accredited MSW and BSW programs for many years) is virtually *entirely* online, save a 2-week on-campus residency in the summer (University of St. Thomas, n.d.).

Many scholars have written entries in the most recent edition of the *Encyclopedia of Social Work,* and published in prominent periodicals, encouraging pursuit of this innovative pedagogical methodology in graduate and undergraduate programs (Coe Regan, 2008; Levin, Whitsett, & Wood, 2013; Ouellette & Westhuis, 2008; Vernon et al., 2009), and one can see no reason why the application of such technology would not be of similar value in doctoral education. In fact, early doctoral-specific research would suggest the appropriateness of online modalities as well for both PhD and DSW education (Bettman, Thompson, Padykula, & Berzoff, 2009; Schoech, 2000; Valentine et al., 1998).

Social work–specific journals have emerged during the past decade, giving increased attention to online education. The *Electronic Journal of Social Work* and *Technology in Social Work Education and Curriculum*, for example, are beginning to include articles on doctoral pedagogy and instruction. Notably, the online revolution offers intriguing opportunities for broadening and extending *access* to doctoral social work education. As we have commented elsewhere,

> With the advent of broadband availability, more powerful processors, secure interactive video transmission, simulcast broadcasting with ITV, versatile web conferencing software, high-end graphics, avatar assisted animation, and sophisticated web-based platforms, the options for online education (and therefore distance learning) today are extensive (Kurzman, 2013, pp. 332–333)

Experience to date would suggest that blended programs, deploying both synchronous (live) and asynchronous (preproduced) components, are likely to be the preferred paradigm. Innovators of online education on the master's degree level emphasize that live chat and Skype technology advances have made a difference in the teaching effectiveness and wider student acceptance of the early technological advances. "Whether by face-to-face interaction via a webcam or the back-and-forth threads of an e-mail chat," Maiden (2013) observed, "the faculty/student interaction that occurs over the course of a semester often achieves an unexpected level of intimacy"

(p. 610). As his fellow pioneers at the University of Southern California have concluded,

> From a social work education perspective, one of the most important [advances] has been the development of synchronous, live interactive technology that has bridged the divide among social work educators and students who are engaged together in online education. . . . Developing asynchronous instruction only or relying solely on Blackboard is an inferior and insufficient approach to online social work course development. (Flynn et al., 2013, pp. 355–356)

For the provision of course instruction, special seminars, peer mentorship, practicum oversight, faculty advising, and dissertation supervision, synchronous options would appear to have the capacity to provide significant added value for doctoral social work programs.

## ACCOUNTABILITY AND ACCREDITATION

The question of accountability increasingly is being mentioned whenever directors of social work doctoral programs come together. As Anastas (2012) stated, "Doctoral programs in social work schools are not accredited by any social work professional organization; rather, they are periodically reviewed internally and in accordance with university-specific or regional accreditation-based standards" (p. 18). The question of why they are not subject to national review is a subject of long-standing debate (Borkowski, 2006; Butler, Rush, & Siman, 1982; Golde & Dore, 2001; Maki & Borkowski, 2006).

> Unlike BSW and MSW programs, social work doctoral education is not accredited by CSWE or any other national organization. Formal external reviews of any given social work doctoral program are generally limited to evaluations conducted by the university at which the program resides. . . . In general, these programmatic reviews reflect the cultural norms of a given university and generally compare the merits of the social work doctoral program with those of comparable doctoral programs across the campus. (Lubben, 2008, pp. 115–116)

In this respect, doctoral programs in social work are an anomaly. Medical schools and law schools, for example, which grant professional doctorates, must undergo national accreditation, and this requirement is the norm for most (if not all) recognized allied health and mental health programs granting the doctoral degree, such as clinical psychology, occupational therapy, audiology, pharmacy, and physical therapy. As recently as 2006, members of a task force appointed by CSWE concluded that "there was a need to examine quality in doctoral education in social work, although there seemed to be little agreement about what the most important problems in quality were" (Anastas, 2012, p. 238). Seven years later, GADE (2013) issued its *Quality Guidelines for PhD Programs in Social Work*, providing specific quality guidelines—including core skills, core supports, core resources, and expected outcomes—without any recommendation regarding how to assess and hence ensure that these outcomes are pursued or achieved. Absent clear standards and oversight, Karger and Stoesz (2003, p. 289) suggested that a danger exists that the proliferation of doctoral programs in underresourced social work schools may deflate the value of the degree.

It would appear ironic to some social work educational leaders that BSW and MSW programs must undergo accreditation (and regular reaccreditation) to maintain the privilege of granting a recognized degree, whereas DSW and PhD programs do not have any such requirement. As noted, GADE makes clear that its guidelines are simply "advisory and aspirational." However, the *Educational Policy and Accreditation Standards* (CSWE, 2008), promulgated by the Council, contain explicit requirements for maintenance of national and legal recognition. In fact, every MSW and BSW program must demonstrate to the Council's Commission on Accreditation that its graduates have generally mastered the requisite 10 Core Competencies and have competence with respect to 41 specified practice behaviors. At the conclusion of her seminal text, Jeane Anastas (2012) aptly observed that, "whereas a new emphasis on learning outcomes in regard to accreditation in social work has been expressed in a competencies orientation at the BSW and MSW levels, those in doctoral education would also do well to consider assessing learning outcomes" (p. 242).

## IMPORTANT ADDITIONAL ISSUES

Although the thoughtful authors of the chapters here in this new book share their views, experiences, findings, and insights, we would emphasize that our discussion presented here merely represents a historical and conceptual framework for the principal prevailing issues in doctoral social work education. The collective strengths and limitations, challenges and achievements, struggles and accomplishments, are far too numerous to mention. This reality, after all, is true for most educational programs in this complex and ever-changing world. We would nevertheless be remiss at this juncture if we were not to make brief mention of several other questions and quandaries facing doctoral social work education. In our judgment they too are worthy of wide discussion and debate. They would include

- Resource requisites for effective doctoral social work education.
- Advantages of the joint social work—social science doctoral degree paradigm.

- Should the topics of ethics and of social justice be expected in a social work doctoral curriculum?
- What are optimum models for doctoral program governance?
- Is the recruitment of racial and ethnic minorities adequate in our doctoral programs?
- What faculty and financial resources are necessary to support students throughout their course of doctoral education?
- Should taking the GRE or MAT be an applicant option or expectation?
- What is the appropriate standard for student mastery of qualitative, quantitative, and mixed method research?
- Should programs be actively measuring the success of graduates in achieving their career goals in research, management, practice, and/or academia?
- What is the role of the philosophy of science in social work PhD programs?
- Is the dissertation the signature pedagogy of doctoral education, or should there be options, such as capstone projects, presentations with publications, and portfolio reviews?
- What should be the distinctive function of DSW degree doctoral education?
- Should there be further consideration of national accreditation of doctoral social work programs?
- Prospectively, what are the appropriate uses of online and distance education formats in social work doctoral education?
- Should we be teaching research-based practice or practice-based research?
- What are the advantages and disadvantages of promoting dual degree options at our universities (e.g., with the DrPH, DDiv, DPA, JD)?
- Do current social work PhD programs prepare graduates appropriately for teaching, and hence for academia?
- What is the proper role of GADE in promoting and supporting doctoral social work education?

We who are involved in and committed to doctoral social work education have many questions to consider, and ultimately many tasks to pursue. This special issue of the *Journal of Teaching in Social Work* has been designed to solicit the advice of many of the wisest scholars committed to the doctoral social work endeavor. It is our hope that, collectively, the several authors here will make a small contribution to offering remedies that will prove to be as comprehensive as the need.

## REFERENCES

Anastas, J. W. (2006). Employment opportunities in social work education: A study of jobs for doctoral graduates. *Journal of Social Work Education, 42*, 195–209. doi:10.5175/JSWE.2006.200400426

Anastas, J. W. (2010). *Teaching in social work: Theory and practice for educators*. New York, NY: Columbia University Press.

Anastas, J. W. (2012). *Doctoral education in social work.* New York, NY: Oxford University Press.

Anastas, J. W., & Kuerbis, A. (2009). Doctoral education in social work: What we know and what we need to know. *Social Work, 54*, 71–81. doi:10.1093/sw/54.1.71

Bettman, J., Thompson, K., Padykula, N., & Berzoff, J. (2009). Innovations in doctoral education: Distance education methodology applied. *Journal of Teaching in Social Work, 29*, 291–312. doi:10.1080/08841230903018397

Borkowski, N. A. (2006). Changing our thinking about assessment at the doctoral level. In P. L. Maki & N. A. Borowski (Eds.), *The assessment of doctoral education: Emerging criteria and new models for improving outcomes* (pp. 11–51). Sterling, VA: Stylus.

Butler, H., Rush, R., & Siman, A. (1982). Evaluation of doctoral programs in social work: Deans' perspectives. In A. Rosen & J. J. Stretch (Eds.), *Doctoral education in social work: Issues, perspectives and evaluation* (pp. 157–166). St. Louis, MO: Group for the Advancement of Doctoral Education in Social Work.

Coe Regan, J. A. (2008). Technology in social work education. In T. Mizrahi & L. Davis (Eds.), *Encyclopedia of social work* (Vol. IV, 20th ed., pp. 217–218). Washington, DC: NASW Press.

Council on Social Work Education. (2008). *Educational policy and accreditation standards.* Retrieved from http://www.cswe.org/File.aspx?id=41861

Council on Social Work Education. (2013). *Statistics on social work education in the United States.* "Doctoral Programs" (36–40). Retrieved from http://www.cswe.org/File.aspx?id=74478

Council on Social Work Education. (2015). *Accreditation statistics.* Retrieved from http://www.cswe.org/Accreditation.aspx

Flynn, M., Maiden, R. P., Smith, W., Wiley, J., & Wood, G. (2013). Launching the virtual academic center: Issues and challenges in innovation. *Journal of Teaching in Social Work, 33*, 339–356. doi:10.1080/08841233.2013.843364

Golde, C. M., & Dore, T. M. (2001) *At cross purposes: What the experiences of doctoral students reveal about doctoral education.* Philadelphia, PA: The Pew Charitable Trust. Retrieved from http://www.phd-survey.org

Group for the Advancement of Doctoral Education in Social Work. (2011). *The doctorate in social work (DSW) degree. Emergence of a new practice doctorate.* Retrieved from http://www.cswe.org/File.aspx?id=59954

Group for the Advancement of Doctoral Education in Social Work. (2013). *Quality guidelines for PhD programs in social work.* Retrieved from http://www.gadephd.org

Group for the Advancement of Doctoral Education in Social Work. (2015). Available at http://www.gadephd.org

Johnson, Y., & Munch, S. (2010). Faculty with practice experience: The new dinosaurs in the social work academy? *Journal of Social Work Education, 46*, 57–66. doi:10.5175/JSWE.2010.200800050

Karger, H. J., & Stoesz, D. (2003). The growth of social work education programs, 1985–1999: Its impact on economic and educational factors related to the profession of social work. *Journal of Social Work Education, 39*, 279–295.

Khinduka, S. (2002). Musings on doctoral education in social work. *Research on Social Work Practice, 12*, 684–694. doi:10.1177/1049731502012005007

Knight, C., & Lagana, M. (1999). The use of a teaching practicum for doctoral students in social work. *Journal of Teaching in Social Work, 18*, 13–22. doi:10.1300/J067v18n01_04

Kurzman, P. A. (2013). The evolution of distance learning and online education. *Journal of Teaching in Social Work, 33*, 331–338. doi:10.1080/08841233.2013.843346

Levin, S., Whitsett, D., & Wood, G. (2013). Teaching MSW social work practice in a blended online learning environment. *Journal of Teaching in Social Work, 33*, 408–420. doi:10.1080/08841233.2013.829168

Lubben, J. E. (2008). Social work education: Doctoral. In T. Mizrahi & L. Davis (Eds.), *Encyclopedia of social work* (Vol. IV, 20th ed., pp. 114–117). Washington, DC: NASW Press.

Maiden, R. P. (2013). Toward the future. *Journal of Teaching in Social Work, 33*, 607–610. doi:10.1080/08841233.2013.846024

Maki, P. L., & Borkowski, N. A. (Eds.). (2006). *The assessment of doctoral education: Emerging criteria and new models for improving outcomes.* Sterling, VA: Stylus.

Munson, C. E. (1996). Should doctoral programs graduate students with fewer than two years of post-MSW practice experience? No! *Journal of Social Work Education, 32*, 167–171.

National Association of Social Workers. (2013). *Advanced practice doctorate* (Unpublished report). Washington, DC: Social Work Policy Institute. Retrieved from http://dsw.socialwork.rutgers.edu/news/nasw-report

O'Neill, J. V. (2000, November). Larger doctoral enrollment sought: Fewer social workers follow path to PhD. *NASW News.* Retrieved from http://www.socialworkers.or/pubs/news/2000/11/phd.htm

Orme, J. (2003). Why does social work need doctors? *Social Work Education, 22*, 541–554. doi:10.1080/0261547032000142652

Ouellette, P. M., & Westhuis, D. (2008). Social work education: Electronic technologies. In T. Mizrahi & L. Davis (Eds.), *Encyclopedia of social work* (Vol. IV, 20th ed., pp. 115–120). Washington, DC: NASW Press.

Pace, P. R. (2013, November 4). Advancing practice doctorate programs. *NASW News, 58*(10), 4.

Proctor, E. K. (1996). Should doctoral programs graduate students with fewer than two years of post-MSW practice experience? Yes! *Journal of Social Work Education, 32*, 161–164.

Raymond, F. B., & Valentine, D. (2001). Doctoral education in social work: Trends and issues. *Arete, 25*, i–iii.

Reisch, M. (2002). The future of doctoral education in the United States: Questions, issues, and persistent dilemmas. *Arete, 26*, 18–28.

Robb, M. (2005, July-August). A deepening doctoral crisis? *Social Work Today, 5*(4), 13–17.

Royeen, C., & Lavin, M. (2007). A contextual and logical analysis of the clinical doctorate for health practitioners. *Journal of Allied Health, 36*, 101–106.

Rutgers University. (n.d.). Doctorate in social work. Retrieved from http://www.socialwork.rutgers.edu/DSW

Schoech, D. (2000). Teaching over the Internet: Results of one doctoral course. *Research on Social Work Practice*, *10*, 467–486.

University of St. Thomas. (n.d.). Doctorate in social work. Retrieved from http://www.stthomas.edu/socialwork/DSW

Valentine, D. P., Edwards, S., Gohagan, D., Hoff, M., Pereira, A., & Wilson, P. (1998). Preparing social work doctoral students for teaching. *Journal of Social Work Education*, *34*, 273–282.

Van Scoy, H. C. (1978). Doctoral education in America: The social work experience. In C. E. Munson (Ed.), *Social work education and practice: Historical perspectives* (pp. 63–84). Houston, TX: Jo Von Books.

Vernon, R., Vakalahi, H., Pierce, D., Pittman-Munke, P., & Adkins, L. (2009). Distance education programs in social work: Current and emerging trends. *Journal of Social Work Education*, *45*, 263–276. doi:10.5175/JSWE.2009.200700081

Zastrow, C., & Bremner, J. (2004). Social work education responds to the shortage of persons with both a doctorate and a professional social work degree. *Journal of Social Work Education*, *40*, 351–358.

# A National Content Analysis of PhD Program Objectives, Structures, and Curricula: Do Programs Address the Full Range of Social Work's Needs?

JAMES DRISKO, CHRISTIE HUNNICUTT, and LAURA BERENSON

*School for Social Work, Smith College, Northampton, Massachusetts, USA*

*The Group for the Advancement of Doctoral Education (GADE) promotes excellence in PhD education in Social Work. GADE's 2013 Quality Guidelines for PhD Programs heavily emphasize preparation for research. Little is known, however, about the details of the contemporary social work PhD program structure and curriculum. Several prior surveys have examined doctoral curriculum requirements, though none was completed in the past 20 years. This content analysis of the 69 U.S.-based, GADE full-member PhD programs offers updated information on program objectives, models, required credit hours, and whether the MSW degree is necessary for admission. The study also summarizes specific curriculum requirements including the number of required courses in research, statistics, practice, policy, philosophy of science, and teaching, along with elective course requirements. Whether research, teaching, and/or practice internships were compulsory and the kinds of dissertations models required for the PhD degree are also reported. Findings show strong emphasis on research and statistics but wide variation in other areas, including teaching and practice. Compared with estimates of labor force needs in the social work profession and academy, it may be that the current emphasis of social work PhD programs does not fully address the core needs of the profession.*

The Group for the Advancement of Doctoral Education in Social Work (GADE) has the primary purpose of promoting excellence in social work doctoral education and asserts that the purpose of PhD education is to prepare stewards of the discipline. Thus, "PhD-trained social work scholars improve the art and science of social work by generating, disseminating, and conserving the knowledge that informs and transforms professional practice" (GADE, 2013, pp. 1–2).

GADE's 2013 *Quality Guidelines for PhD Programs in Social Work* document strongly emphasizes knowledge development through both research and teaching. Emphasis on social work practice, and the balanced practitioner/researcher model of PhD education that was included in the earlier 1992 and 2003 GADE *Quality Guidelines*, has been deleted. The current (GADE, 2013) document states that PhD students should be able to "critically analyze theories, practices, policies, and research" and "should be able to understand the relations among social work education, research, and practice" (p. 2). Being able to *do* direct social work practice, or to *do* policy practice, is not highlighted.

Further, GADE does not argue for (or recommend) that an MSW degree should be required for admission to PhD studies in social work. Advanced expertise in research is put forward as the main objective of social work PhD programs, rather than developing additional expertise in direct social work practice or policy practice. Although the current GADE statement therefore represents a move toward standardization among PhD programs in social work, some variations in PhD programs may be evident, and intentional. Notably, Shore and Thyer (1996) argued against individuals without an MSW degree being accepted for doctoral degrees in social work. They contended that allowing non-MSWs to gain advanced social work degrees is harmful to the profession.

Jeane Anastas (2012) noted that "information on doctoral education and social work is limited" (p. 5). Indeed, the published literature on doctoral education in social work is small. Although the Council on Social Work Education (CSWE) provides annual data on student enrollment and graduation rates, it does not address program structure or curriculum content. Indeed, no recent study of doctoral program structure and curriculum content is available. This content analysis offers what may be the first contemporary data on the structure and content of GADE member PhD programs in the United States.

## PRIOR STUDIES OF THE DOCTORAL CURRICULUM IN SOCIAL WORK

Royse (1980) examined the program descriptions and curriculum content of 32 social work doctoral programs (as found in their 1977 admissions materials) and reported that 84% of programs required research or statistics content, with little difference between DSW (88%) and PhD (80%) granting programs. Seventy-two percent of programs required policy content. Practice content was required by only 44% of the programs.

Rubin and Davis (1981) surveyed the 33 doctoral programs being offered at the time regarding core curriculum content. They found that 91% (30) programs had required research courses, of which 85% focused on research methods and 70% addressed statistics. Only three programs (9%) had a research practicum. A full 88% had required courses on policy, 64% on practice, and 33% on administration. Twenty-seven percent of social work doctoral programs in 1981 had a practice concentration. Only 24% mandated courses on education or teaching, and only 6% had a required teaching practicum. A decade later, Fraser, Jenson, and Lewis (1991) again examined doctoral research course content. They found that the 47 doctoral programs in social work at the time *all* required research content. Somewhat later, Anastas and Congress (1999) finally called for greater attention specifically to philosophy of science and to a range of suitable epistemologies.

Although data on doctoral education in social work is quite limited (and now dated), similar themes still appear. Scholars frequently criticize doctoral education for being too "social science oriented" and insufficiently attentive to "professional social work" (Anastas, 2012, p. 3), or, being caught "between research and teaching" (p. 16). Several calls have been made for placing greater emphasis in social work PhD programs on educating teachers (Chipungu, 2012; Fraser, 2012; Pryce, Ainbinder, Werner-Lin, Browne, & Smithgall, 2011). Zastrow and Bremner (2004) pointed to a need for more social workers with both a professional *and* a doctoral degree to teach practice and to guide practice research. Given the less than universal content on practice found in both Royse's (1980) and Rubin and Davis's (1981) surveys, there may continue to be a tension between research and practice in social work doctoral education. Hence, it is not clear whether current PhD programs in the United States meet the knowledge, practice, and hiring needs of the social work profession.

It is also worth noting that very little study of PhD comprehensive examinations has been undertaken. Furstenberg and Nichols-Casebolt (2001) examined the general merit of comprehensive examinations but did not systematically explore the forms of exam actually in use by doctoral programs. Similarly, the kinds of research, teaching, and practice internships offered by contemporary PhD programs have not been very carefully examined.

Closely allied professions, such as psychology (American Psychological Association, 2013), communications (Schiappa, 2009), and health care professions (University of California, San Francisco, n.d.), have consistently emphasized the importance of *both* educating researchers *and* educating highly skilled advanced practitioners at the PhD level. In these professions, research, practice, clinical mentorship, and classroom teaching all receive emphasis as needed in order to educate stewards of these professions.

The social work profession has sought very consciously to increase its research infrastructure and expertise over the past 20 years but may have shifted away from addressing the needs of the larger profession in the process of this pursuit, including research talent among educators. More balanced attention to serving the needs of the profession as a whole via doctoral education may now be needed.

## THE HIRING OUTLOOK IN SOCIAL WORK AND SOCIAL WORK EDUCATION

The U.S. Bureau of Labor Statistics (BLS; 2013) noted that the employment of social workers is expected to grow by 25% from 2010 to 2020. This is faster than the BLS average prediction for all occupations. Although BLS defines social workers without regard to specific professional education, they stated that most of this growth will be in direct practice. Therefore, the need for doctoral-level social workers to educate a growing practice workforce in the coming years seems clear. Simply put, expertise in *doing* direct social work practice and in *doing* policy practice appears to be a primary educational need in the early 21st century.

CSWE (2013) statistics show that the vast majority of university-based social work education is directed to professional preparation at the baccalaureate and the master's levels. The need to educate students at these levels suggests a need for an expanded cohort of doctoral-level graduates, with a range of knowledge and skills that extend beyond research alone, to prepare for faculty positions in the CSWE-accredited programs that will educate them.

## DOCTORAL EDUCATION AND THE HIRING NEEDS OF THE ACADEMY

Khinduka (2002) stated that there is a continuing undersupply of doctoral graduates in social work. Mackie (2013) reported that there are about 300 published faculty job announcements for social work positions each year. Further, CSWE (2013, p. 15) statistics show that there were 307 doctoral graduates in 2012 and an average of 319 graduates per year between 2008 and 2012. However, surveys also show that only about half of these doctoral graduates will seek employment in the academy (Anastas, 2012). Consequently, the undersupply of doctoral graduates appears likely to continue. Anastas (2006) studied faculty recruitment advertisements and found the stated areas of expertise sought among candidates for appointment were practice (58%), social policy (22%), research (22%), human behavior in the social environment (18%), and fieldwork (10%). The need for practice expertise among new faculty hires in social work cannot be ignored.

This study provides current information on the program objectives and required content of GADE full-member PhD programs in social work (not including those in candidacy or DSW programs) in the United States. Such information may guide future discussions about the purposes and directions of social work doctoral education. The data also can inform the profession regarding how well current doctoral programs are educating graduates to meet our profession's full range of hiring needs.

## THE STUDY GOALS

This descriptive endeavor examined each doctoral program's (a) stated objectives, (b) use of full-time or part-time (or both) program models, (c) number of required credit hours for graduation, (d) whether an MSW degree was required for admission, and (e) the typical length of each PhD program and the maximum allowed years to completion. The study also addressed (f) the number of required courses in research, statistics, practice, policy, philosophy of science, and teaching, and (g) the number and types of required elective courses. Our pursuit further sought to address whether (h) a research internship, (i) a teaching internship, and (j) a practice internship was required. To document student achievement, (k) the forms of comprehensive exams required (if any) and (l) the forms of dissertations models each program allowed also were examined.

## METHODS

A content analysis (Krippendorf, 2013) was completed to determine PhD program objectives, structure, and curriculum characteristics. As noted, the study sample included all American-based GADE full-member PhD programs as of August 2013. (GADE currently states that it has more than 80 member programs, but at the time of this study [spring 2013] there were 70 full-member PhD programs in the United States. In addition, there were some member programs located outside the United States, several PhD programs "in candidacy," and a few DSW program members as well.) One PhD program (Tulane) was a GADE member but was not accepting new applications. Hence, all the 69 operating U.S. GADE full-member PhD programs were the study's sample. The two independent-member (non-GADE) PhD programs were excluded. DSW degree programs not addressed by GADE's (2013) *Quality Guidelines for PhD Programs* also were intentionally excluded, as the study focus was solely on PhD programs.

The researchers visited and copied the websites of all the 69 operating social work doctoral programs in the United States to create the core data set. In all cases but three, the online data proved very detailed and complete. (It is possible that the online data may have been somewhat outdated, because specific dates on some materials were absent.) Material from the three programs with limited or incomplete online content was obtained by e-mail. In addition, telephone calls were made by the researchers to clarify some ambiguities in program content. As always, there was some missing or equivocal data with respect to a few variables due to program variation and differences in labeling.

The three researchers initially read the program materials of five settings for training purposes and to determine the posttraining level of interrater reliability. The posttraining alpha coefficient was $\alpha = .94$. A second reader later reviewed another eight programs read by others, documenting a high level of interrater reliability as analysis continued ($\alpha = .96$). Unclear or missing content and rounding error led to some totals not fully representing all 69 programs or reaching a 100% value.

The data analysis plan is descriptive in nature. The modal value was used because the obtained responses generated highly skewed distributions for which the mode seemed more appropriate than a mean. The mean also would be impacted by outlier high values and by numerous zero values found on several items. The range of responses also is reported to summarize the variation found.

# FINDINGS

## PhD Program Objectives

There is wide variation in the stated objectives of social work PhD programs in United States. Yet there is also strong consistency and emphasis on research, statistics, development of knowledge, and production of scholars. All online program descriptions ($n = 69$) included "educating researchers" or "knowledge development." A full 80% ($n = 55$) also embraced "educating competent scholars." Slightly less than half (49%, $n = 34$) emphasized academic or professional leadership. Forty-six percent ($n = 32$) included "educating teachers," whereas 33% ($n = 23$) emphasized "policy planning." Only 13% ($n = 9$) stated a goal of educating for administration.

Some PhD programs specifically contrasted their doctoral program objectives with direct or clinical practice. Seventeen percent ($n = 12$) stated that they "did *not* offer advanced clinical training," whereas 14% ($n = 10$) specifically noted that they *did* offer "advanced practice training." The nature of practice training varied widely. For example, Columbia University and Widener University each offer an academic track specific to practice. Wayne State University and Smith College both offer a practice focus and mandate a doctoral practicum. Practice courses more often focused on theories of practice, knowledge for practice, or the evidence base of practice, rather than on conducting direct practice.

## Program Structures

Fifty-five percent ($n = 38$) of U.S. PhD programs in social work offer both full-time and part-time program options. Another 36% ($n = 25$) were full-time only. Only 7% ($n = 5$) were *solely* part-time programs. Credits required for graduation ranged from 36 plus dissertation to 89 plus dissertation. (The modal number of required credits for graduation was 48 plus dissertation.) Time to degree completion was listed typically as ranging from 3 to 7 years, with a modal value of 4 to 5. The maximum time allowed for PhD degree completion ranged from 7 years to "10 years plus revalidation." The modal value for time allowed to PhD degree completion was 7 years.

Only 23% ($n = 16$) of social work PhD programs specifically required an MSW degree for admission. A few of these programs also required some post-MSW experience in practice or policy, whereas others merely recommended such experience. A full 33% ($n = 23$) of programs had no explicit degree requirements for PhD admission. A few required "an MSW in progress" or that "non-MSWs must take two MSW courses"; some only mandated an MSW degree for the clinical track. Overall, 77% ($n = 53$) of social work PhD programs did not require an MSW degree for admission.

## Required Courses

All 69 (100%) social work programs required research courses (see Table 1). The actual number of required research courses ranged from two to six. The modal number of required research courses was three. All 69 programs also required courses in statistics, with a range from one to six and a modal value of two. Because some programs combined research and statistics content within a single course, our analysis counted fractions of courses that then were tallied to identify more distinct research and statistics course counts. About one third of the PhD programs had a requisite qualitative research course, and many more offered qualitative research electives as options.

Dissertation proposal seminars were the next most frequently required PhD course. Eighty-six percent of programs ($n = 59$) required enrollment in dissertation proposal development seminars. Sixty-two percent ($n = 44$) required policy courses, with a range of zero to four courses and a mode of two. Slightly less than half of the programs (49%, $n = 34$) required participation in teaching or social work education courses, ranging from zero to two, interestingly with a mode of zero. However, elective courses on teaching often were available where education courses were not required.

**TABLE 1** Required Courses by Specific Content Area

| Course focus | N (%) Requiring courses | Range of required courses | Modal no. of required courses |
|---|---|---|---|
| Research | 69 (100%) | 2–6+ | 3 courses |
| Statistics | 69 (100%) | 1–6 | 2 courses |
| Electives | 69 (100%) | 2–5 | 2 courses |
| Dissertation Proposal Seminar | 59 (86%) | 0–3 | 1 course |
| Policy | 44 (62%) | 0–4 | 2 courses |
| Teaching/Education | 34 (49%) | 0–2 | 0 courses |
| Philosophy of Science/ Epistemology | 27 (39%) | 0–2 | 0 courses |
| Professional Writing | 27 (39%) | 0–2 | 0 courses |
| Social Theory | 21 (30%) | 0–2 | 0 courses |
| Practice | 19 (28%) | 0–6 | 0 courses |
| HBSE | 15 (22%) | 0–5 | 0 courses |

*Note.* Modal values are reported since many of the distributions were highly skewed and both high outliers and multiple zero values undermine the clarity of mean values. $N = 69$. These are all the full membership GADE programs in the United States (other than Tulane University, which was suspended after the Katrina flood). HBSE = human behavior and social environment.

Thirty-nine percent ($n = 27$) of programs required courses on epistemology or on the philosophy of science, with a range of zero to two courses and a mode of zero. Thirty-nine percent ($n = 27$) mandated courses on professional writing, with a range of zero to two courses and a mode of zero. Thirty percent ($n = 21$) required social theory courses, with a range of zero to two courses and a mode of zero. Twenty-eight percent ($n = 19$) offered requisite practice courses, with a range of zero to six courses and a mode of zero. Finally, 22% of programs required HBSE courses, with a range of zero to five courses and again a mode of zero. In sum, considerable variation in required course content is evident in tandem with consistent core requirements in research methods and statistics.

## Elective Courses

All 69 programs required the completion of electives as part of the PhD course of study, frequently as a vehicle for allowing students to develop an area of specialization. The number of elective courses required for the degree ranged from two to five with a modal score of two. Electives course requirements often were "cognates," or courses taken in other disciplines or professional schools. The use of cognate courses versus social work specific courses varied widely, as did their content. Elective courses on ethics or values were the most frequent option, followed (in descending order) by social theory, integrative seminars, writing courses, organizational theory, "cross-national or global perspectives," grant writing, leadership, economics, information technology, and oppressed or vulnerable populations.

## Required Internships

Fifty-eight percent ($n = 40$) of the programs required research internships or practica (see Table 2). Another 10% ($n = 7$) simply encouraged research internships. It was unclear from program documents whether students who serve as research assistants are viewed as being involved in research internship. The availability of research assistant opportunities was often noted in program documents, of course, as contingent on the availability of funding. Specifically, in 46% ($n = 32$) of programs, internships were stated as funded, but one third of these also were listed as "competitive" or "when available." Such statements make an overall analysis of the availability of research internships quite challenging. It may well be that the 58% figure is low.

On the other hand, only 23% ($n = 16$) of these programs required teaching internships. Another 13% ($n = 9$) listed teaching internships as "optional" or "by request." Once again, it was difficult to determine whether other teaching opportunities were regularly available to these doctoral students. Online program documents that address funding one's education suggest that many students participate in paid teaching assistantships or teach courses in their 3rd and later years of PhD education. In fact, 68% ($n = 47$) of programs indicate that teaching opportunities are available at some point during the student's PhD course of study. However, program documents do not clearly specify the degree of oversight and mentoring provided during these teaching opportunities.

Only 3% ($n = 2$) of social work PhD programs required practice internships. None were funded, although one program provided financial aid for purchasing additional supervision during the internship. An additional 3% ($n = 2$) of PhD programs required an internship solely for students who did not have an MSW degree.

**TABLE 2** Required PhD Internships

| Required internship type | $N$ (%) requiring | Optional internship | Funded |
|---|---|---|---|
| Research | 40 (58%) | 7 (10%) | 32 (46%) One third were "competitive" or "when available" |
| Teaching | 16 (23%) | 9* (13%) | Unclear—many as paid instructor |
| Practice | 2 (3%) | 0† (0%) | 1 work-study |

*Note.* $N = 69$.
*47 (68%) indicate that some form of teaching opportunity is available.
†Another 2 (3%) require a practice internship only for students without an MSW degree to compensate for the lack of an MSW level internships. This is not, however, a formal requirement of the PhD course of study *per se.*

## Comprehensive Examinations

Eighty-eight percent ($n = 61$) of the programs required comprehensive examinations. The other 12% ($n = 8$) either did not explicitly require a comprehensive examination or simply did not address it in their online program materials. Three models of examination were apparent: 55% ($n = 38$) of the full 69 programs required the traditional written exam, addressing one or more questions, followed by an oral exam; 19% ($n = 13$) required a manuscript intended for professional publication; and 10% ($n = 7$) mandated completion of papers (or sections) of the student's dissertation proposal. The other 4% ($n = 3$) stated that they required a comprehensive examination but did not specify its format or content. The reported timing of comprehensive examinations ranged from "after year one" to "after all courses." The modal timing of the comprehensive exam was "after year two."

## The Dissertation

All of the PhD programs (100%, $n = 69$) appear to accept the tradition dissertation model, although in a few cases the nature of the dissertation was not clearly explicated. Twenty-four percent ($n = 17$) also allow the "three publishable paper" dissertation option or a "varied format." Descriptions of supports for dissertations appeared to vary widely in the materials available online. The beginning of dissertation work was described as ranging from "early in studies" to "after all courses are completed." The modal timing for the start of dissertation work was "year three." General grading expectations for the dissertation were posted, but specific details of the dissertation process (and supports for it) were highly variable in the program materials.

## DISCUSSION

### Program Objectives

The focus of these PhD programs appears to be in sync with their most commonly stated program objective: to prepare researchers and scholars. These objectives also are consistent with one of two main areas emphasized in GADE's (2013) *Quality Standards for PhD Programs*. Most social work PhD programs prioritized the development of scholars, which would seem to emerge as an area of clear strength for social work PhD programs. However, fewer than half of the programs also emphasized academic or professional leadership, and only 46% underscored educating teachers in their program objectives—even though teaching is the second main area emphasized in GADE's (2013) *Quality Guidelines for PhD Programs*. It could be argued that preparing teachers and leaders for the profession as a whole should be more clearly and widely emphasized in the objectives and required courses of PhD-level social work education.

Notably, one of the least emphasized areas was education for advanced social work practice. Indeed, more programs specifically disavowed a focus on advanced practice education than offered it (17% vs. 14%). Perhaps this limited attention to policy and to practice is meant to affirm the sound level of preparation provided by social work baccalaureate and master's degree programs. PhD courses of study, however, seek to enhance and elaborate upon the prior education of students in the area of research and theory. Hence, it is not clear why PhD-level education in social work practice, administration, and policy would not be equally beneficial to students, to clients, and to the profession. Attention to core content areas beyond research may be deserving of even greater and more consistent attention in the program objectives of social work PhD education.

## Program Structure

Contemporary social work PhD programs offer a mix of full- and part-time options, which provide a good range of options for prospective applicants. It is not clear from these data if financial aid and opportunities for research, teaching, and practice internships vary by full- versus part-time status. Biegel and Yoon (2014) stated that the increase in full-time PhD programs over the past 20 years offers students more opportunities for involvement in research. This may well be so, but 36% of these social work PhD programs offer only full-time program options. Given these findings, how the choice of full- versus part-time options shapes the content and financial viability of a student's PhD educational opportunities deserves additional, detailed study.

As noted, credits required for PhD completion varied widely. Some of this variation may be accounted for by semester hour versus quarter hour differences that were not always clearly stated online. The modal requirement of 48 credits (plus dissertation) appears comparable to allied professions. A quick online review of credit requirements for a PhD in psychology revealed a range of 32 to 94 credit hours (though some included credit for work toward a master's degree), plus dissertation, nursing PhD requirements ranged from 47 to 60 credit hours beyond master's degree, plus dissertation. Social work's credit expectations for the PhD degree therefore appear roughly consistent with similar professions.

## Requiring the MSW Degree

Seventy-seven percent of social work PhD programs do not require an MSW degree for admission. If, as GADE (2013) stated, completion of an MSW signifies solid foundational knowledge of social work as a professional practice, this overwhelming element of flexibility may undermine the value orientation, practice skill, and overall social work competence of PhD graduates. Not requiring an MSW degree does provide a mechanism for bringing talented individuals into the profession but would suggest the possibility of less acculturation and socialization to the profession for individuals. The PhD programs that require additional courses for students without an MSW degree clearly seek to make up for these differences. Yet not all social work PhD programs have additional requirements for students who do not hold an MSW degree. Further, it is not clear that additional courses alone would adequately help PhD students fully understand the application of social work's person-in-environment perspective, understand social work values, refine specific skill sets, or assure that they will gain an understanding of the challenges and complexities of teaching or doing social work practice.

The decision to allow non-MSWs into social work PhD programs also has licensing implications, as 41 states appear to allow licensure as a professional social worker with only a PhD degree (no MSW) (Edwards, Holmes, & Rittner, n.d.). Protecting the public and providing quality services are just as important goals as expanding PhD programs' applicant pools. Higher education institutions need to seek talent within the accrediting requirements; hence, GADE (and social work's other educational and professional organizations) should engage in further discussion on this topic.

## Increased Active Involvement in Research and Teaching

It is not surprising that social work PhD programs emphasize education in research methods and statistics. *All* these programs required research courses, which represents an expansion since Royse's (1980) report 35 years ago and which is consistent with Fraser et al.'s (1991) somewhat more recent findings. The PhD programs appear to provide in-depth research education via required and elective research and statistics courses, often tailored to subspecialty areas and fields of practice. Required research internships have grown dramatically since Rubin and Davis found back in 1981 that only three programs offered such opportunities. Fifty-eight percent of programs now require research internships, with many of these being paid opportunities. Nevertheless, this may mean that many PhD graduates *will not* engage in hands-on research experience beyond their dissertation work. Perhaps research internships should be made available to *all* social work PhD students in order to ensure the preparation of skilled stewards of the discipline.

Only 46% of these programs stated that educating teachers was a central PhD program objective. Although required teaching or education courses are now part of 49% of social work PhD curricula, up from 25% in 1981 (Rubin & Davis), it is not clear that this meets GADE (2013) quality standard for competence in teaching for PhD graduates. Although 68% of programs state that they offer teaching opportunities, it is not clear that these are actually pedagogical opportunities for guided student learning about teaching. Only 23% of programs required teaching internships and another 13% offered similar but optional internship opportunities. This is an improvement, of course, over the 6% of programs offering teaching internship opportunities in 1981, but nonetheless seems quite limited. Educating and developing skilled social work educators logically should be an even greater part of all required PhD programs in order to meet rapidly expanding labor market needs.

## Reduced Required Content in Other Content Areas

In 1981, Rubin and Davis found that 88% of social work doctoral programs required courses on social policy. In 2013, however, only 62% required policy courses, although many other programs offered such elective options. In 1981, 33% of programs mandated courses in administration, whereas in 2013 only 16% had such a requirement. Attention to administration and community organization practice perhaps should also be expanded as opportunities for PhD-level social work study.

In 1981, Rubin and Davis found that 64% of social work doctoral programs required practice courses, and a full 27% had doctoral practice concentrations. In 2013, required practice courses were found in only 28% of social work PhD programs and merely 3% required practice internships. Advanced-level practice education clearly has declined rapidly as social work has increased its emphasis on the education of researchers. Yet practice expertise is needed to develop new knowledge, implement evidence-based findings, lead agencies, prepare field liaisons, and provide high-quality supervision. Consequently, it appears logical that social work's PhD programs should continue to support practice knowledge and expertise.

GADE (2013) has formally deleted the practitioner/researcher paradigm of PhD education, which it supported from 1992 until 2012. Yet the combination of practice and research expertise continues to be a valid and useful approach to PhD education in social work, especially in this era of evidence-based practice. Such a practitioner/researcher doctoral model is common, even routine, in closely allied professions (American Psychological Association, 2013; University of California, San Francisco, n.d.).

It is clear that social work PhD education programs have markedly increased their emphasis over the past two decades on the education of researchers. They also have somewhat increased attention to the education of teachers to meet the growing needs of higher education institutions. Nonetheless, it is unclear if social work PhD programs are optimally meeting the broader hiring and service needs of the social work profession for expertise in policy, practice, and administration. Maintaining balanced attention to the full range of needs of the profession may require modest modifications in PhD education. GADE, and other social work organizations, must use data-driven approaches to ensure that the education and practice needs of the entire profession are met fully by its PhD programs. This study provides one source of data for such review and professional dialogue.

## FUNDING

This research was supported by a grant from the Brown Foundation Clinical Research Institute of the Smith College School for Social Work.

## REFERENCES

American Psychological Association. (2013). *Preparing professional psychologists to serve a diverse public*. Retrieved from http://www.apa.org/pi/lgbt/resources/policy/diversity-preparation.aspx

Anastas, J. (2006). Employment opportunities in social work education: A study of jobs for doctoral graduates. *Journal of Social Work Education, 42*, 195–209. doi:10.5175/JSWE.2006.200400426

Anastas, J. (2012). *Doctoral education in social work*. New York, NY: Oxford University Press.

Anastas, J., & Congress, E. (1999). Philosophical issues in doctoral education in social work: A survey of doctoral program directors. *Journal of Social Work Education, 35*, 143–153.

Biegel, D., & Yoon, S. (2014). Social work education: Research. In C. Franklin (Ed.), *Encyclopedia of social work online* (21st ed., pp. 1–6). New York, NY: Oxford University Press. doi:10.1093/acrefore/9780199975839.013.618

Bureau of Labor Statistics. (2013). *United States occupational outlook handbook, 2012-13 ed., Social workers*. Retrieved from http://www.bls.gov/ooh/community-and-social-service/social-workers.htm

Chipungu, S. (2012, April). *Preparing educators: How doctoral programs can prepare BSW level educators; How BSW programs can support scholars*. Paper presented at the GADE Annual Conference, Portland, OR.

Council on Social Work Education. (2013). *2012 statistics on social work education in the United States*. Alexandria, VA: Author.

Edwards, R., Holmes, J., & Rittner, B. (n.d.). *The doctorate in social work (DSW) degree: Emergence of a new practice doctorate*. Retrieved from http://ww.gadephd.org/Portals/0/docs/DSWGuidelines2011t.pdf

Fraser, M. (2012, April). *Preparing educators: How doctoral programs can prepare BSW level educators; How BSW programs can support scholars*. Paper presented at the GADE Annual Conference, Portland, OR.

Fraser, M., Jenson, J., & Lewis, R. (1991). Training for research scholarship in social work doctoral programs. *Social Service Review, 65*, 597–613. doi:10.1086/603877

Furstenberg, A.-L., & Nichols-Casebolt, A. (2001). Hurdle or building block: Comprehensive examinations in social work doctoral education. *Journal of Teaching in Social Work, 21*, 19–37. doi:10.1300/J067v21n01_03

GADE. (2013). *Quality guidelines for PhD programs in social work*. Retrieved from http://gadephd.org/Portals/0/docs/GADE%20quality%20guidelines%20approved%204%2006%202013%20%282%29.pdf

Khinduka, S. (2002). Musings on doctoral education in social work. *Research on Social Work Practice, 12*, 684–694. doi:10.1177/1049731502012005007

Krippendorf, K. (2013). *Content analysis: An introduction to its methodology.* Newbury Park, CA: Sage.

Mackie, P. (2013). Hiring social work faculty: An analysis of employment announcements. *Journal of Social Work Education, 49,* 133–141.

Pryce, J., Ainbinder, A., Werner-Lin, A., Browne, T., & Smithgall, C. (2011). Teaching future teachers: A model workshop for doctoral education. *Journal of Teaching in Social Work, 31,* 457–469. doi:10.1080/08841233.2011.601941

Royse, D. (1980). Social work doctoral education programs: A consumer's eye view. *Journal of Education for Social Work, 16,* 43–48. doi:10.1080/00220612.1980.10778506

Rubin, A., & Davis, R. (1981). The elusive doctoral curriculum: A dilemma for the social work profession. *Areté, 6*(3), 1–9.

Schiappa, E. (2009). *Professional development during your doctoral education.* Washington, DC: National Communications Association. Retrieved from http://comm.umn.edu/assets/pdf/ProfDevBK.pdf

Shore, B., & Thyer, B. (1996). Should non-MSWs earn the social work doctorate? A debate. *Journal of Teaching in Social Work, 14,* 127–145. doi:10.1300/J067v14n01_08

University of California, San Francisco. (n.d.). *Doctoral program in health professions education.* Retrieved from http://meded.ucsf.edu/radme/doctoral-program-health-professions-education

Zastrow, C., & Bremner, J. (2004). Social work education responds to the shortage of persons with both a doctorate and a professional social work degree. *Journal of Social Work Education, 40,* 351–358.

# Current Issues in Social Work Doctoral Education

HARRIET GOODMAN

*Silberman School of Social Work, Hunter College, and*
*The Graduate Center of the City University of New York, New York, New York, USA*

*The purpose of doctoral programs in social work is to prepare research-scientists who contribute to knowledge that guides professional practice and educators competent to teach new cohorts of social work practitioners. In grooming stewards of the profession, doctoral programs also must prepare their graduates to support the larger contemporary needs of the profession, including its long-standing commitment to economic and social justice, particularly during a period of increasing inequality. The newly adopted 2013 GADE Quality Guidelines provide the building blocks for evaluation and renewal for social work doctoral programs. These include knowledge of social work as a discipline, research and scholarship, teaching, and aspirational outcomes for students, each of which is critically examined within the current context of U.S. doctoral programs and the status of the social work profession.*

## INTRODUCTION

Doctoral programs in social work prepare students to generate and disseminate new knowledge that will serve to guide the social work enterprise. They are also the major source of faculty members for bachelor's and master's degree social work programs. Graduates seek to apply their doctoral studies in various ways—as academic scholars, independent researchers, organizational leaders, policymakers, and advocates (Anastas, 2012a; Jenson, 2008; Valentine et al., 1998). However, the extent to which social work doctoral programs prepare students to support the larger contemporary needs of the profession still remains an unanswered question and is a topic of considerable discussion and debate (Abell & Wolf, 2003; Anastas, 2006; Anastas & Kuerbis, 2009; Fong, 2012, 2014; Jenson, 2008; Johnson & Munch, 2010; Mayadas, Smith, & Elliott, 2001; Ortega & Busch-Armendariz, 2014; Pollio, 2012; Reisch, 2002, 2013; Valentine et al., 1998; Zastrow & Bremner, 2004). Much of this debate centers on the preparation of doctoral students to navigate social work's dual emphasis on direct practice and social reform in their roles as research scientists and teachers.

Unlike BSW and MSW programs, which prepare students for practice, PhD and DSW programs are research degrees. Consequently, doctoral programs are not subject to Council on Social Work Education (CSWE) accreditation. However, beginning in 1992 and again in 2002, the Group for the Advancement of Doctoral Education (GADE), the membership organization of the most highly regarded social work doctoral programs in the United States, developed guidelines for doctoral programs to address concerns about their quality. The GADE membership approved revised *Quality Guidelines* for PhD programs at the organization's 2013 annual meeting (Harrington, Petr, Black, Cunningham-Williams, & Bentley, 2014). The new *Guidelines* are consistent with the Carnegie Initiative on the Doctorate's (CID) conception of doctoral education being to prepare students as stewards of the discipline (Golde & Walker, 2006; Walker, Golde, Jones, Bueschel, & Hutchings, 2008). That is, PhD-trained social work scholars should improve the art and science of social work by "generating, disseminating, and conserving the knowledge that informs and transforms professional practice" (Harrington et al., 2014, p. 282). The revised guidelines not only reflected CID principles but also incorporated survey results from 416 doctoral students, faculty, and administrators and drew on a number of publications referred to in this article (Anastas, 2012a; Brekke, 2012; Fong, 2012). As such, the *Guidelines* represent a consensus from a broad constituency about current standards for member programs. The GADE *Guidelines* propose building blocks for doctoral studies that programs can use to develop, renew, and improve social work PhD programs. These include knowledge of social work as a discipline and profession, research and scholarship, teaching, and aspirational outcomes for students (Harrington et al., 2014). With adequate structures and resources, PhD programs are charged with preparing their students as researchers, teachers, and community and organizational leaders—and when they assume these roles to conserve the professional values identified with social work.

The concept of "stewardship" put forth by the CID suggests that doctoral education preserve the professional disciplines by fostering renewal and creativity while it inculcates future scholars in the knowledge, practices, and values of their respective fields (Golde & Walker, 2006; Walker et al., 2008). Stewards not only are prepared to develop new knowledge but also reflect on existing theories, research, texts, and historical context to determine what constitutes the essence of their discipline. As teachers, stewards are responsible for identifying what is essential to teach and then communicating that specialized knowledge both within the classroom and to practitioners, cultural communities, and the larger society (Golde & Walker, 2006; Walker et al., 2008).

In this context, few social workers assume stewardship, and stakeholders will depend on a small proportion of them who pursue doctoral studies to teach and conduct research. The 2% of American MSW graduates who go on to obtain the PhD in social work (Anastas, 2006) bear the responsibility to provide essential professional leadership as knowledge generators and transmitters with particular attention to contemporary policy shifts and their effects on how social workers actually deliver services.

A long-standing issue that confounds stewardship in social work is the rift between scientific inquiry and practice (Orcutt, 1990; Tsang, 2000). Within the contemporary political and social climate, the implications of the practice/research divide within U.S. social work doctoral education are particularly profound (Horton & Hawkins, 2010). While advancing the principles and methods of science *in* the profession, social work doctoral education must maintain professional values and the transmission of practice knowledge as it develops *for and from* practitioners working in the field. Consequently, integration of both research and practice at the micro- and macrolevels is essential for realizing stewardship in social work. However, achieving this goal may be problematic when there is a chasm between research priorities and broader professional needs (Belcher, Pecukonis, & Knight, 2011; Epstein, 2009, 2011; Tsang, 2000); in reality, bridging the division between practice and research has been particularly problematic in social work during the first decade of the 21st century (Mor Barak & Brekke, 2014).

Although most American doctoral programs strive for scholarship and research that will drive or serve practitioner needs and are firmly embedded in social work's core mission and values, academic, institutional, and investigator priorities often are shaped by the preferences of major grant-making entities (Anastas, 2012a; Corvo, Chen, & Selmi, 2011; Howard, 2011; Thyer, 2011). Problems that social workers experience in the field do not necessarily guide social work research. In addition, research support accrues disproportionately to a limited number of institutions and investigators (Corvo et al., 2011). For example, Corvo et al.'s (2011) analysis of National Institutes of Health research grants to schools of social work between 1993 and 2005 found that 13 of the most highly ranked universities received 75% of National Institutes of Health funding. The pursuit of federal funding raises other issues, as well; it can narrow the scope of social work research, and investigators may avoid controversial topics central to the concerns of the profession (Corvo et al., 2011; Peck, 2009). Of equal concern, as other institutions strive to mirror the profile of these schools, the social work research enterprise "may be drawn toward a certain narrow epistemology that may undermine more critical aspects of the profession" (Corvo et al., 2011, p. 231).

Certainly, all doctoral programs must prepare scholars for current and future methodological and analytic advances both as scientists and research-informed pedagogues. Nevertheless, if U.S. doctoral programs narrow their objectives; limit themselves to particular methods and subjects of scholarly inquiry, and proceed to prepare educators, scholars, and policymakers accordingly, they may be diverging from the profession's long-standing commitment to a larger social vision. Social work doctoral programs may risk encouraging emerging scholars to distance themselves from unfolding social needs and isolating themselves from the universal experiences of social work practitioners and the marginalized groups they frequently serve (Ortega & Busch-Armendariz, 2014; Reisch, 2013).

Current trends, such as acceleration in the production of (and access to) knowledge and new ways in which academic work and the wider world interact, are areas of concern (Walker et al., 2008). These features anticipate the inevitability of rapidly accelerating changes (Kurzweil, 2000) that will call on nimble professional leaders to respond to new trends as the century progresses. Stewardship during this period of rapid technological change, and dramatic political, economic, and environmental challenge, calls on doctoral graduates to make significant contributions to research-informed policy and practice. This is the only way they will be able to advance the work of practitioners for the turbulent times in which they will be working.

This article assumes that for social work to increase its influence in the amelioration of social problems and the promotion of positive social change, it must address the role doctoral education has in preserving long-standing professional values. The doctoral enterprise is responsible for preparing researchers to contribute to knowledge and educators competent to teach new cohorts of social work practitioners. Programs therefore need to equip doctoral graduates to analyze social problems in ways that position the profession to achieve progressive social policy objectives. However, if their research pursuits hinge on the primacy of particular methods and a market-driven production of scholarship, their research will risk evading the most pressing social problems our society confronts today (Ortega & Busch-Armendariz, 2014; Reisch, 2013). Similarly, as educators, PhD students will need to be keenly aware of the "swamps" and "messes" social workers routinely encounter in practice (Lester, 2004, p. 764) if they are to address the concerns their students bring to the classroom.

## TRENDS IN DOCTORAL EDUCATION

The first American social work doctoral program opened in 1915 at Bryn Mawr College, offering a PhD in social research; in 1920, the University of Chicago initiated a PhD in social administration. Both programs emanated from historic social service settings such as settlement houses, and they were driven by the power of professional leadership for progressive social action. The earliest social work doctoral offerings focused on research and theory germane to social policy and research, as opposed to direct practice (Orcutt, 1990). Social work doctoral programs increased over time. In 1950, nine programs offered a doctorate in social work, and by 1960 the number had increased to 16. The 1980s saw a 20% increase in such programs, and in the 1990s there was even more substantial growth, with 53 programs granting doctorates by 1993 (Anastas & Kuerbis, 2009). As of this writing, membership listed on the GADE website includes 75 U.S. programs, eight Canadian programs, and one Israeli program that offer the PhD; in addition, four U.S. programs are in development. Four GADE member programs currently offer the DSW in addition to the PhD (GADE, n.d.).

Although the earliest programs offered the PhD, around 1950 schools began to offer a professional doctorate, the DSW, which identified with social work as a profession. Consequently, Catholic University, which had offered the PhD when it opened its program in 1934, changed from the PhD to the DSW in 1948 along with Smith College and the University of Pennsylvania (Baldi, 1971). The DSW programs that predominated between the 1950s and 1990s included practice- and research-based study, whereas the PhD followed a scientist-practitioner model (Barsky, Green, & Ayayo, 2014). As early as 1975, Crow and Kindelsperger (1975) suggested that the PhD should be reserved for knowledge building, whereas the DSW would serve as an advanced practice degree. Accordingly, the PhD would prepare students for producing research and the DSW would produce advanced micro- and macropractitioners. These authors recognized the flexibility essential to a profession's evolving and complex societal functions. After all, not only does social work concern itself with developing, conserving, and transforming knowledge, but its portfolio of practice also includes service delivery, social policy formation, and the pursuit of social justice and social change (Anastas, 2012a).

Nonetheless, the 1990s saw the full embrace of the PhD and abandonment of the DSW, which frequently paralleled the increasing dominance of the research component of social work doctoral education (Austin, 1983; Crow & Kindelsperger, 1975; Edwards, 2011). As a result, current PhD curricula in social work have placed increasing emphasis on epistemology, research methods, and social work science (Abell & Wolf, 2003; Brekke, 2012; Fong, 2012, 2014; Harrison & Thyer, 1988; Jenson, 2008).

Doctoral education contributed to the quest for professionalization in social work research, education, and practice (Reeser & Epstein, 1990), continuously shaped by periods of ascendancy and erosion of the welfare state and the accompanying political, economic, and ideological forces (Reisch, 2002). Whether granting PhDs or DSWs, social work has always looked to doctoral education for increased professional status. This theme persists today, reified by the preference at a growing number of universities for programs that emphasize research in the form of advanced quantitative methodological and analytic skills (Jenson, 2008). Noting the improved image the PhD and empirical research has projected, David Austin wrote, "Indeed, the current concerns about the distinctions between the PhD and the DSW, and the redesign of DSW programs as PhD programs, attest to the power of the symbols associated with empirical research in establishing status within a university" (Austin, 1983, p. 371).

An attempt to prepare students for clinical practice and leadership, firmly grounded in research, recently appeared in the emergence of four new DSW programs in the United States. Although offering the DSW as the professional doctorate, and the PhD as the research doctorate, has wide acceptance in many other countries, it is a new and developing trend in the United States. Some suggest that the reemergence of the DSW is a response to recent competition from aggressively advertised online and institute-based options. The DSW programs offered in GADE-affiliated schools, however, make practice doctorates available to social workers willing to pay for their convenience and the prestige of programs offered through high-status, accredited universities (Anastas & Videka, 2012).

To some, the DSW represents a vestige of a time when the profession had lower status, and for those who entered social work doctoral studies in the 1960s and 1970s, best left in the past. Still, it is undeniable that the first decade of the 21st century has seen a revival of the DSW for clinical practice and leadership (Anastas & Videka, 2012), and most recently a program to prepare students as teachers (University of St. Thomas, 2015). Currently, the four DSW programs listed on the GADE website include the University of Pennsylvania, the University of Tennessee, Rutgers University, and the University of St. Thomas/St. Catherine University. A review of their program websites suggests that DSW programs target students who are working professionals. Two programs accommodate students through course modules in weekend or summer study and two others through distance learning technology. This pattern supports Crow and Kindelsperger's (1975) prediction that PhD programs could serve the knowledge-building component of doctoral education and the DSW could be reserved for advanced practitioners. We discuss these programs later in relation to doctoral studies and social work education.

## Doctoral Education and the Preparation of Research Scholars

In developing revised *Quality Guidelines*, the GADE Task Force referred to the national movement promoting the science of social work and to the work of John Brekke (2012) and Rowena Fong (2012) in particular (Harrington et al., 2014). However, the section of the guidelines on research/scholarship does not explicitly mention "science," although it does call for a significant investment in the development of research competency among PhD students. Although the "science of social work" is a topic of considerable interest in doctoral education, it is an evolving and contested conceptualization. Claims that social researchers are doing more intervention service systems and translational research that are "driving research standards to new levels of sophistication" (Fong, 2014, p. 607) provide one rationale for promoting examination of "social work as science" in doctoral education. This path leads to the question of whether "social work as science" should inform the curricula of all U.S. doctoral programs, even though it is evident that some PhD program directors' dominant view of social work is as a profession where the application (not the production) of research is paramount (Anastas, 2014; Fong, 2014). Nonetheless, it is likely that programs heavily identified with research in the logical positivist tradition advocate social work as a research-based "science" (Brekke, 2012, 2014; Fong, 2012) and support the argument that the dominant role of doctoral education is to create scientists who generate knowledge through research.

Moving past the rhetoric associated with the "science of social work" debate, Pollio (2012) operationalizes that construct for doctoral education, stating, "The purpose of the doctoral education process is not to train scientists, but to uniquely train social work scientists" (p. 538). He drafted principles for research curricula and dissertation research to achieve that purpose. In the first instance, Pollio asserted that training social work scientists requires students to be familiar with social work as a profession and have knowledge of the field. He identified specific areas of research training that include development of multiple, complementary skills; courses in the philosophy of science; and the integration of theory. In addition, he argued that preparation of doctoral students as scientists requires sophistication in multiple methods and the ability "to design robust, real-world research and also be able to develop sophisticated, complex designs" (p. 539). This proposal has the potential to embrace divergent views of social work as practice and social work as science.

Unfortunately, many American doctoral students and faculty mentors currently conceptualize and conduct research at a fair distance from the context, problems, and aspirations of contemporary practice (Aisenberg, 2008; Anastas, 2014). Some of the most prominent U.S. faculty scholars do their research under conditions that contrast markedly with present agency-based work environments (Fong, 2012). Regrettably, this encourages a one-way relationship between research and practice (Anastas, 2012b, 2014; Johnson & Munch, 2010) that reinforces a secondary "consumer" role for practitioners in their relationships with researchers (Katz, 2006). Even doctoral students note that their programs are more aligned with a "culture of academia" and that their practice experiences and interests are devalued; some clearly "wish there could be a way to bring together practice and research" (Anastas, 2012a, p. 44).

Without educational leadership that recognizes and resists these trends, and is willing to collaboratively integrate research and practice, the relevance of emergent inquiry for the dilemma of agency-based practice is questionable (Pollio, 2012; Robb, 2005). Consequently, a question currently vexing American doctoral educators is how to connect the information deficits of contemporary practice with knowledge that sustains the ambitions of a profession historically grounded in practice and informed by a mission of social justice.

It is not possible to discuss unifying practice and research without considering the need for PhD students to become methodological pluralists, with competence in an array of methods, as opposed to researchers with "an obsession with methodological rigor" in the positivist tradition (Rolfe, 1995, p. 105). Feilzer's (2010) statement that "pragmatism [enables] researchers to enjoy the complexity and messiness of social life and revive a flagging sociological imagination" (p. 14) parallels the contention that unitary research approaches that privilege experimental design are often incompatible with the needs the social work profession has to excavate the many layers in which practice is embedded. Equally problematic is the enduring bifurcation of the constructivist and postpositivist models. Some assert that offering separate qualitative and quantitative research method courses implies that students must take a position in the paradigm debate (Feilzer, 2010). The current crop of 21st-century scholars is still a product of the wars that appear to bedevil doctoral education with their unitary commitment to one approach or the other (Tashakkori & Creswell, 2008). At the same time, the complex problems that proliferate in the practice arena require examining research problems from multiple methodological perspectives (Feilzer, 2010; Morgan, 2014).

In response to this dilemma, there is a strong argument for doctoral social work education that promotes methodological pluralism, that is, a collection of scientific approaches that are compatible with practice-relevant research (Anastas, 2012b, 2014; Cornish & Gillespie, 2009; Feilzer, 2010; Oktay, 2012). This paradigm, which might be called "methodological humility," contends that there is no one best method but instead urges researchers to determine which method (or combinations of methods) best addresses real-world questions. An important feature of the "pragmatic paradigm" is its attention to the social and political context of knowledge development and utilization. This approach has the potential to bridge the "practice versus research divide."

In this discourse, it is essential that practice research incorporates problems important to a variety of stakeholders (Anastas, 2012b), not simply those which elite researchers—or their funding sources—deem important. Anastas (2012b) specifically pointed to Epstein's clinical data mining (Epstein, 2010, 2011) as a means to engage practitioners in the systematic collection and analysis of agency data to answer practice-generated questions. She also identified community-based participatory action research (Torre, Fine, Stoudt, & Fox, 2012) as an empowerment tool for engaging community partners in research, and as being highly compatible with the social justice mission of the profession. When doctoral students have the ability to work within a broad array of methods and across disciplines, it enriches their research.

## Doctoral Education and the Preparation of Social Work Faculty

GADE stipulates that the province of social work education is to serve the discipline and its research tradition. Consequently, doctoral education prepares academic scholars to make significant contributions both to the scientific literature and to social work education (Harrington, Petr, Black, Cunningham-Williams, & Bentley, 2014). Most doctoral students expect that their primary employment will be as faculty members, where they will both teach and conduct research (Anastas, 2012a, p. 171). This aspiration is important to the field, because MSW and BSW programs presently face shortages of doctoral-prepared faculty, and particularly those who can teach practice courses within the CSWE's Education Policy and Accreditation Standards (Anastas, 2006, 2012a; Barsky et al., 2014; Mackie, 2013). The current CSWE standards require that "faculty who teach social work practice courses have a master's degree in social work from a CSWE-accredited program and at least two years of practice experience" (CSWE, 2012, Standard 3.3.1). When students move quickly from MSW programs to doctoral studies their practice experience may be limited, and some may not have worked in the field post-MSW at all.

Although a topic less addressed in tenure track faculty hiring, faculty members also need to be able to teach from a social justice perspective, for which they may not have received preparation in their course of doctoral study (Hudson, Shapiro, Moylan, Garcia, & Derr, 2014). The CSWE Education Policy and Accreditation Standards calls on MSW programs to instruct students to "understand the forms and mechanisms of oppression and discrimination and advocate for human rights and social and economic justice" (CSWE, 2012, Standard 2.1.5). However, doctoral programs, which do not undergo CSWE accreditation, may not prepare students to teach this content. In a study of the role of educators in promoting a social justice orientation, one faculty member reported, "If you are going to make social justice a core part of the profession, there needs to be a core doctoral training course in social justice, and there isn't (Not anywhere I've been.)" (Funge, 2011, p. 85).

In 2006, Anastas studied trends in employment opportunities for doctoral graduates in social welfare. She found that in the 2001–2002 academic year, more faculty positions were available than social work doctoral graduates to fill them. In other words, there was (and continues to be) an undersupply of qualified doctoral graduates to meet the need of accredited social work education programs (Anastas, 2006, 2012a). This shortfall is occurring in the face of a proliferation of newly accredited BSW and MSW programs and has persisted 10 years after Anastas's original study. The urgent need for PhD graduates to teach when on tenure track lines is evident in reports from BSW and MSW program deans and directors (Barsky et al., 2014; Mackie, 2013). Even so, announcements for people seeking to fill faculty positions expect both more pregraduation scholarship and teaching experience on the part of applicants for those positions. They call not only for the PhD but also the MSW, 2 or more years of post-MSW practice experience, teaching experience as a lead instructor, a clear teaching philosophy, and often a willingness to teach both bachelor's- and master's-level students (Anastas, 2006, 2012a).

Recent advertisements for faculty positions circulated on the GADE listserv also indicate a strong preference for applicants with successful grant-making activity, a well-formulated research trajectory, and curricula vitae that demonstrate ample peer review presentations and publications. Among the "On the Market" announcements distributed widely on both the GADE and the National Association of Deans and Directors listservs, job seekers at one university must supply both a research and a teaching statement in addition to a curriculum vitae. The growing emphasis on grant writing, publication, and research grant achievement, while students are pursuing the PhD, further reinforces their separation, if not their divorce, from the world of practice.

Critically, the efficient movement of researcher-scholars from doctoral programs to full-time academic positions both reveals and promotes the misfit between pressing practice instructional needs of bachelor's- and master's-level programs and the skill sets of recent doctoral graduates who cannot possibly approximate a scholar-teacher-practitioner model or even acquire a social work license (Belcher et al., 2011). Takamura (2008) pointed out that the integration of the classroom with changing field conditions continually challenges master's-level social work programs. In that respect, students who move directly from MSW to PhD programs are likely to be unfamiliar with the sober and stressful realities of contemporary practice that MSW students confront daily in their field placements.

Exacerbating the situation further, faculty members often are able to buy out teaching time with funds in their research grants (Belcher et al., 2011).

This reality suggests a trend in some institutions toward hiring full-time faculty with strong research potential and finding other ways of accommodating the need for a full complement of classroom instructors. The most common solution is through hiring adjunct instructors who have direct experience of practice but may have little research knowledge or respect for the value of research (Zastrow & Bremner, 2004). In addition, because of the poor supply of PhD graduates with practice experience, some social work programs are recruiting untenured "clinical instructors" who are not expected to develop a portfolio of research and publication (Barsky et al., 2014). The trend toward hiring non-tenure-track clinical faculty to teach practice courses is evident in the increasing number of these positions posted on the GADE listserv.

If schools of social work leave practice instruction to adjuncts and non-tenure-track clinical instructors, they rely on people, meritorious as they may be, without a persistent link to the life of the programs that hire them (Belcher et al., 2011; Johnson & Munch, 2010). Hiring "clinical" faculty members to fill the practice experience gap is a problematic solution, because it creates a two-tier system in the academic setting and denigrates practice in the eyes of students whose ambitions overwhelmingly are for careers as practitioners. It should be noted that the downgrading of classroom instruction in colleges and universities is a problem across academic institutions (Katz, 2006). However, it is even more critical in BSW and MSW programs, because what occurs in the classroom and the field must inform each other. Practice-relevant research must serve as a bridge at that intersection. Professors with the ability to bring research-mindedness to the classroom promote theory and empirical study as the basis for action among their students.

In the past, doctoral programs in social work have been agnostic regarding whether curricula should include explicit preparation for an academic role (Karger & Stoesz, 2003). Some (Valentine et al., 1998) advocated strongly that doctoral students should receive preparation for teaching and asserted that graduates would otherwise be unprepared to provide high-quality education for MSW and BSW students. Consequently, some doctoral programs provide courses or seminars in pedagogy and promote authentic teaching opportunities for pre- and postdoctoral students in anticipation of their aspirations to become educators. Currently, slightly more than half of all social work doctoral programs require students to take a course on teaching, although less than one fourth of those courses address the need to use evidence in their teaching (Lind, Maynard, & Albright, 2015). Although coursework in the theory and practice of teaching is worthwhile, it cannot substitute for instruction in the design and delivery of a course. Inevitably, courses in pedagogy provide technique, not experience.

GADE's 2013 *Quality Guidelines* recognize that knowledge alone is inadequate for preparing doctoral students as educators. Core expertise and skills in this area now cover knowledge of adult learning theory as well as specific issues instructors in social work programs are likely to encounter, such as addressing issues of diversity and ethical dilemmas that will emerge in class. The *Guidelines* also call for programs to provide doctoral students the opportunity to design and teach a course that is a part of the accredited social work curriculum (Harrington et al., 2014).

Currently one advantage proffered for the newly minted DSW programs is their potential to support the production of practitioner-educator-scholars who will have considerable practice experience (Edwards, 2011). However, as suggested earlier, many have reservations about this "solution," because many MSW and BSW programs already have a de facto two-tier professorate—those with the PhD who pursue scholarship and those hired as adjuncts or "clinical" faculty, who are not expected to conduct research. However, it is far too early to comment on the impact these programs will have on social work education.

## CONCLUDING THOUGHTS

The question of whether American doctoral education has become so narrow that it cannot support broad-based research or prepare postsecondary educators is an issue of great concern throughout academia (Katz, 2006; Wilson, 2010). The professorate and the universities that employ them are "increasingly disrespectful of both the larger intellectual contours of the disciplines and the needs of future teacher-scholars" (Katz, 2006, p. B10). Another widespread complaint is that whatever the discipline, the most opportunistic and entrepreneurial researchers are the most highly rewarded, although they may primarily serve the needs of a narrow research community. In this environment, teaching, nontraditional scholarship, and community service are less valued (Katz, 2006; Peck, 2009). In other words, doctoral programs in social work may join a long list of American academic disciplines that privilege particular methodologies and streams of funded research and publication, primarily in high-impact journals. This pattern leaves aside a diverse array of alternative inquiry and places less value on teaching. This tendency also raises the question of whether present patterns in contemporary doctoral education in social work are consistent with longstanding professional social work values.

The implications of current academic priorities are particularly stark for social welfare, given the compelling need for critical examination of complex, layered trends in a field where PhD graduates will work as research-practitioners, academics, policymakers, and organizational leaders. In addition, the movement toward scientist-scholars, as opposed to practice-research-scholars, suggests that issues closest to contemporary practice may go unstudied. Reisch (2013) contended that neo-liberalism has encouraged the "commodification of knowledge" (p. 720). Because the scientist-scholar model most often applies a unitary approach to research, elevating experimental design, it also marginalizes alternative methodologies that would be more appropriate in order to study the multifaceted problems social workers of all stripes encounter in practice.

Beginning in the 1990s, the National Institute of Mental Health established Task Force on Social Work Research (1991) sought ways to track MSW students efficiently for doctoral study, and research-intensive universities organized their PhD programs so this could occur. Practices such as combined MSW/PhD programs and recruiting students immediately upon receipt of the MSW, supporting students as research assistants on faculty grant-funded projects, and enabling students to use faculty mentor data secondary as a platform for dissertation research have become characteristics of the most highly ranked doctoral programs. Students associated with these programs have an advantage in establishing early research, publication, and grant-making profiles. They also are fortunate if they have independent teaching opportunities as students rather than merely acting as teaching assistants for their mentors. Although highly competitive when on the academic job market, such doctoral graduates often lack practice experience. As a result, they confound the efforts of search committees seeking faculty members who can both achieve tenure and teach credible courses in practice and in human behavior.

The accelerating pace of evolving social problems suggests the need for immediacy of response on the part of social work scholars. We should keep in mind McLuhan and Fiore's (1967) insightful reflection on the difficulty in keeping pace with unfolding events: "We look at the present through a rear view mirror. We march backwards into the future" (p. 74).

We have questioned whether social work doctoral programs are preparing students to adequately address the broader needs of the profession. An important responsibility of graduates with PhDs in the discipline is to inform social work as a practice. Doctoral education should prepare researchers whose scholarship strengthens practice and who will educate aspiring practitioners. It is out of complexity and contradiction that innovation occurs. An important contribution of the revised GADE *Guidelines* is their challenge to social work doctoral program faculty and directors to respond to these needs as their programs evolve.

# REFERENCES

Abell, N., & Wolf, D. (2003). Implementing intervention research in doctoral education: Maximizing opportunities in training for outcome evaluation. *Journal of Teaching in Social Work, 23*, 3–19. doi:10.1300/J067v23n01_02

Aisenberg, E. (2008). Evidence-based practice in mental health care to ethnic minority communities: Has its practice fallen short of its evidence? *Social Work, 53*, 297–306. doi:10.1093/sw/53.4.297

Anastas, J. W. (2006). Employment opportunities in social work education: A study of jobs for doctoral graduates. *Journal of Social Work Education, 42*, 195–209. doi:10.5175/JSWE.2006.200400426

Anastas, J. W. (2012a). *Doctoral education in social work*. New York, NY: Oxford University Press.

Anastas, J. (2012b). From scientism to science: How contemporary epistemology can inform practice research. *Clinical Social Work Journal, 40*, 157–165. doi:10.1007/s10615-012-0388-z

Anastas, J. W. (2014). The science of social work and its relationship to social work practice. *Research on Social Work Practice, 24*, 571–580. doi:10.1177/1049731513511335

Anastas, J. W., & Kuerbis, A. N. (2009). Doctoral education in social work: What we know and what we need to know. *Social Work, 54*, 71–81. doi:10.1093/sw/54.1.71

Anastas, J. W., & Videka, L. (2012). Does social work need a 'practice doctorate'? *Clinical Social Work Journal, 40*, 268–276. doi:10.1007/s10615-012-0392-3

Austin, D. M. (1983). The Flexner myth and the history of social work. *Social Service Review, 57*, 357–377. doi:10.1086/644113

Baldi, J. J. (1971). Doctorates in social work, 1920–1968. *Journal of Education for Social Work, 7*, 11–22. doi:10.1080/00220612.1971.10671859

Barsky, A., Green, D., & Ayayo, M. (2014). Hiring priorities for BSW/MSW programs in the United States: Informing doctoral programs about current needs. *Journal of Social Work, 14*, 62–82. doi:10.1177/1468017313476772

Belcher, J., Pecukonis, E., & Knight, C. (2011). Where have all the teachers gone? The selling out of social work education. *Journal of Teaching in Social Work, 31*, 195–209. doi:10.1080/08841233.2011.562103

Brekke, J. (2012). Shaping a science of social work. *Research on Social Work Practice, 22*, 455–464. doi:10.1177/1049731512441263

Brekke, J. S. (2014). A science of social work, and social work as an integrative scientific discipline: Have we gone too far, or not far enough? *Research on Social Work Practice, 24*, 517–523. doi:10.1177/1049731513511994

Cornish, F., & Gillespie, A. (2009). A pragmatist approach to the problem of knowledge in health psychology. *Journal of Health Psychology, 14*, 800–809. doi:10.1177/1359105309338974

Corvo, K., Chen, W., & Selmi, P. (2011). Federal funding of social work research: High hopes or sour grapes? *Social Work, 56*, 225–233. doi:10.1093/sw/56.3.225

Council on Social Work Education. (2012). *Education policy and accreditation standards (2012 revision)*. Retrieved from http://www.cswe.org/Accreditation/2008EPASDescription.aspx

Crow, R. T., & Kindelsperger, K. W. (1975). The PhD or the DSW? *Journal of Education for Social Work, 11*(3), 38–43. doi:10.1080/00220612.1975.10778699

Edwards, R. L. (2011). *The doctorate in social work (DSW) degree: Emergence of a new practice doctorate: Report of the task force on the DSW degree convened by the Social Work Leadership Forum*. Retrieved from http://www.gadephd.org/documents/DSWGuidelines2011t.pdf

Epstein, I. (2009). Promoting harmony where there is commonly conflict: Evidence-informed practice as an integrative strategy. *Social Work in Health Care, 48*, 216–231. doi:10.1080/00981380802589845

Epstein, I. (2010). *Clinical data-mining: Integrating practice and research*. New York, NY: Oxford University Press.

Epstein, I. (2011). Reconciling evidence-based practice, evidence-informed practice, and practice-based research: The role of clinical data-mining. *Social Work*, *56*, 284–288. doi:10.1093/sw/56.3.284

Feilzer, M. Y. (2010). Doing mixed methods research pragmatically: Implications for the rediscovery of pragmatism as a research paradigm. *Journal of Mixed Methods Research*, *4*, 6–16. doi:10.1177/1558689809349691

Fong, R. (2012). Framing education for a science of social work: Missions, curriculum, and doctoral training. *Research on Social Work Practice*, *22*, 529–536. doi:10.1177/1049731512452977

Fong, R. (2014). Framing doctoral education for a science of social work: Positioning students for the scientific career, promoting scholars for the academy, propagating scientists of the profession, and preparing stewards of the discipline. *Research on Social Work Practice*, *24*, 607–615. doi:10.1177/1049731513515055

Funge, S. P. (2011). Promoting the social justice orientation of students: The role of the educator. *Journal of Social Work Education*, *47*, 73–90. doi:10.5175/JSWE.2011.200900035

Golde, C. M., & Walker, G. E. (Eds.). (2006). *Envisioning the future of doctoral education: Preparing stewards of the discipline*. San Francisco, CA: Jossey-Bass.

Group for the Advancement of Doctoral Education in Social Work. (n.d.). *US members*. Retrieved from http://www.gadephd.org/Membership

Harrington, D., Petr, C. G., Black, B. M., Cunningham-Williams, R., & Bentley, K. J. (2014). Quality guidelines for social work PhD programs. *Research on Social Work Practice*, *24*, 281–286. doi:10.1177/1049731513517145

Harrison, D. F., & Thyer, B. A. (1988). Doctoral research on social work practice: A proposed agenda. *Journal of Social Work Education*, *24*, 107–114.

Horton, E. G., & Hawkins, M. (2010). A content analysis of intervention research in social work doctoral dissertations. *Journal of Evidence-Based Social Work*, *7*, 377–386. doi:10.1080/15433710903344066

Howard, M. O. (2011). Harmful effects of federal research grants: A rejoinder. *Social Work Research*, *35*, 9–10. doi:10.1093/swr/35.1.9

Hudson, K. D., Shapiro, V. B., Moylan, C., Garcia, A., & Derr, A. S. (2014). Teaching note—Infusing social justice into doctoral programs of social welfare: An incremental approach. *Journal of Social Work Education*, *50*, 559–567.

Jenson, J. M. (2008). Enhancing research capacity and knowledge development through social work doctoral education. *Social Work Research*, *32*, 3–5. doi:10.1093/swr/32.1.3

Johnson, Y. M., & Munch, S. (2010). Faculty with practice experience: The new dinosaurs in the social work academy? *Journal of Social Work Education*, *46*, 57–66. doi:10.5175/JSWE.2010.200800050

Karger, H. J., & Stoesz, D. (2003). The growth of social work education programs, 1985-1999: Its impact on economic and educational factors related to the profession of social work. *Journal of Social Work Education*, *39*, 279–295.

Katz, S. N. (2006). What has happened to the professoriate? *Chronicle of Higher Education*, *53*(7), B8–B11.

Kurzweil, K. (2000). *The age of spiritual machines*. New York, NY: Penguin.

Lester, S. (2004). Conceptualizing the practitioner doctorate. *Studies in Higher Education, 29*, 757–770. doi:10.1080/0307507042000287249

Lind, K. S., Maynard, B. R., & Albright, D. L. (2015, January). *Pedagogical training in social work doctoral programs: An analysis of curricula and syllabi.* Paper presented at the 19th Annual Convention of the Society for Social Work Research, New Orleans, LA.

Mackie, P. F.-E. (2013). Hiring social work faculty: An analysis of employment announcements with special focus on rural and urban differences and 2008 EPAS implications. *Journal of Social Work Education, 49*, 733–747.

Mayadas, N. S., Smith, R. I., & Elliott, D. (2001). Social groupwork in doctoral programs: Implications for social work practice and education. *Journal of Teaching in Social Work, 21*, 175–194. doi:10.1300/J067v21n01_11

McLuhan, M., & Fiore, Q. (1967). *The medium is the message: An inventory of effects.* New York, NY: Bantam.

Mor Barak, M. E., & Brekke, J. S. (2014). Social work science and identity formation for Doctoral scholars within intellectual communities. *Research on Social Work Practice, 24*, 616–624. doi:10.1177/1049731514528047

Morgan, D. L. (2014). Pragmatism as a paradigm for social research. *Qualitative Inquiry, 20*, 1045–1053. doi:10.1177/1077800413513733

Oktay, J. S. (2012). *Grounded theory.* New York, NY: Oxford University Press.

Oktay, J. S., Jacobson, J. M., & Fisher, E. (2013). Learning through experience: The transition from doctoral student to social work educator. *Journal of Social Work Education, 49*, 207–221. doi:10.1080/10437797.2013.768108

Orcutt, B. A. (1990). *Science and inquiry in social work practice.* New York, NY: Columbia University Press.

Ortega, D., & Busch-Armendariz, N. (2014). Elite knowledge or the reproduction of the knowledge of privilege: Social work doctoral education. *Affilia, 29*, 5–7. doi:10.1177/0886109913517162

Peck, S. L. (2009). Science suffers when getting a grant becomes the goal. *Chronicle of Higher Education, 55*(7), A42.

Pollio, D. E. (2012). Response: Training doctoral students to be scientists. *Research on Social Work Practice, 22*, 537–541. doi:10.1177/1049731512442573

Reeser, L. C., & Epstein, I. (1990). *Professionalism and activism in social work.* New York, NY: Columbia University Press.

Reisch, M. (2002). The future of doctoral education in the United States: Questions, issues, and persistent dilemmas. *Areté, 26*(2), 18–28.

Reisch, M. (2013). Social work education and the neo-liberal challenge: The US response to increasing global inequality. *Social Work Education: The International Journal, 32*, 715–733. doi:10.1080/02615479.2013.809200

Robb, M. (2005). A deepening doctoral crisis? *Social Work Today, 5*(4), 13.

Rolfe, G. (1995). Playing at research: Methodological pluralism and the creative researcher. *Journal of Psychiatric and Mental Health Nursing, 2*, 105–109. doi:10.1111/j.1365-2850.1995.tb00150.x

Takamura, J. C. (2008). The graduate social work dean: Roles and reflections. In L. H. Ginsberg (Ed.), *Management and leadership in social work practice and education* (pp. 377–392). Alexandria, VA: Council on Social Work Education.

Tashakkori, A., & Creswell, J. W. (2008). Editorial: Envisioning the future stewards of the social-behavioral research enterprise. *Journal of Mixed Methods Research*, *2*, 291–295. doi:10.1177/1558689808322946.

Task Force on Social Work Research. (1991). *Building social work knowledge for effective services and policies—A plan for development*. Austin: University of Texas, School of Social Work.

Thyer, B. A. (2011). Harmful effects of federal research grants. *Social Work Research*, *35*, 3–7. doi:10.1093/swr/35.1.3

Torre, M., Fine, M., Stoudt, B. G., & Fox, M. (2012). Critical participatory action research as public science. In H. Cooper (Ed.), *APA handbook of research methods in psychology, volume 2. Research designs* (pp. 117–184). Washington, DC: American Psychological Association.

Tsang, A. K. T. (2000). Bridging the gap between clinical practice and research: An integrated practice-oriented model. *Journal of Social Service Research*, *26*(4), 69–90.

University of St. Thomas. (2015). About the doctorate in social work. Retrieved from http://www.stthomas.edu/socialwork/dsw/about/

Valentine, D. P., Edwards, S., Gohagan, D., Huff, M., Pereira, A., & Wilson, P. (1998). Preparing social work doctoral students for teaching: Report of a survey. *Journal of Social Work Education*, *34*, 273–282.

Walker, G. E., Golde, C. M., Jones, L., Bueschel, A. C., & Hutchings, P. (2008). *The formation of scholars: Rethinking doctoral education for the twenty-first century*. San Francisco, CA: Jossey-Bass.

Wilson, R. (2010). The ivory sweatshop: Academe is no longer a convivial refuge. *Chronicle of Higher Education*, *56*, B28–B32.

Zastrow, C., & Bremner, J. (2004). Social work education responds to the shortage of persons with both a doctorate and a professional social work degree. *Journal of Social Work Education*, *40*, 351–358.

# Patterns and Trends of Canadian Social Work Doctoral Dissertations

DAVID W. ROTHWELL, LUCYNA LACH, ANNE BLUMENTHAL,
and BREE AKESSON
*School of Social Work, McGill University, Montreal, Quebec, Canada*

*The first social work doctoral program in Canada began in 1952. Relatively recently, the number of programs has grown rapidly, doubling in the past 10 years to 14 programs. Despite the expansion there is no systematic understanding of the patterns and trends in doctoral research. In this study we review 248 publicly available dissertations from 2001 to 2011. We find that most dissertations are qualitative and descriptive in nature with a relatively low percentage focusing on intervention. We compare findings with other dissertation studies and raise critical questions about the knowledge base of social work in Canada.*

There are currently 39 schools of social work that are members of the Canadian Association for Social Work Education (CASWE) offering undergraduate and graduate social work programs; of these, 14 offer doctoral programs.[1] Compared to programs in the United States, where the first doctoral program was established in 1917 (Reisch, 2002), Canadian programs are young but growing rapidly. The first Doctor of Social Work program was developed at the University of Toronto in 1952; it remained the only such program in Canada for more than 30 years, until additional programs opened at Wilfrid Laurier University and Laval University in 1987

---

[1] Nine of these 14 schools are members of the Group for the Advancement of Doctoral Education in Social Work: McGill University, Memorial University, University of Montreal, Universite Laval, University of Calgary, University of Manitoba, University of Toronto, University of Windsor, and Wilfrid Laurier University.

(Shera, 2003). Doctoral education, however, has expanded rapidly in the past decade, with the number of such programs doubling to the present count of 14. This substantial increase is a reflection of enhanced government funding to universities for graduate-level education, as well as a commitment by academic leaders to allocate resources toward doctoral-level education in order to expand intellectual leadership (Council of Ontario Universities, 2012). Although the curricula vary across programs, the overarching goal is to produce graduates capable of independent research.

There currently is no formal mechanism for these programs to reflect on the landscape of doctoral education in Canada. Although a number of them are members of the U.S.-based Group for the Advancement of Doctoral Education in Social Work, there is no equivalent forum in Canada. To our knowledge, just three articles have been written on doctoral social work education in Canada. Key pedagogical questions have been studied in other countries but have not yet been addressed in Canada. For example, what are the most commonly studied social problems? What research methods are being employed, and therefore taught? To what extent is social work engaging in systematic inquiry of social interventions? Considering the rapid growth of doctoral social work programs in the country, it is imperative to know more in order to help social work develop its intellectual and disciplinary identity.

The first study of doctoral social work in Canada came in the form of a mail survey conducted by James Gripton, a member of what was then called the Faculty of Social Welfare, University of Calgary (Gripton, 1982). His was a survey of Canadians with doctoral education in social work ($n = 64$), 48% of whom were educated in the only doctoral program in Canada at the time, the University of Toronto. (The remaining respondents obtained their degrees outside Canada.) Gripton documented their student experience while enrolled in their respective doctoral programs, employment and income trends before and after graduation, scholarly productivity, and demographic characteristics. One limitation of that study was that it did not distinguish between those who received their doctoral education in Canada and those educated in other countries; therefore, findings do not apply exclusively to Canadian doctoral programs.

In 1991, Shankar Yelaja, Dean of the Faculty of Social Work at Wilfrid Laurier University, described the four doctoral programs that existed at the time and the challenges facing doctoral social work education in Canada (Yelaja, 1991). One of the critical issues he identified was a tension between the extent to which doctoral education should focus on advanced practice skills as opposed to research training. This debate seems to have been resolved, as none of the current doctoral programs emphasizes advanced practice skills. Instead, all programs are research intensive and require a dissertation that makes a unique contribution to the substantive field of inquiry.

Twelve years later, Wes Shera, then Dean of the Faculty of Social Work at the University of Toronto, surveyed the seven programs in Canada at the time (Shera, 2003). Under ideas for improving doctoral programs, two themes emerged in the analysis (in order): more financial support for students, and the need to adapt to student needs while maintaining high standards. Among 10 additional individual comments, Shera reported a need to improve resources for innovative, independent research and a need to achieve a better balance between qualitative and quantitative modalities of research. Although the aforementioned studies lay an important foundation for understanding the evolution and issues related to doctoral education in Canada, to date we have no systematic understanding of the nature and patterns of doctoral social work scholarship in Canada.

The quality and content of doctoral education in social work has been studied by a number of researchers in the United States (Anastas & Congress, 1999; Anastas & Kuerbis, 2009; Horton & Hawkins, 2010; Maynard, Vaughn, & Sarteschi, 2012), the United Kingdom (Lyons, 2002; Scourfield & Maxwell, 2010), Taiwan (Shek, Lee, & Tam, 2007), and Sweden (Dellgran & Höjer, 2001, 2012). Two additional U.S.-based reviews have focused specifically on qualitative dissertations (Brun, 1997; Gringeri, Barusch, & Cambron, 2013). Collectively, these studies have used a variety of methods (e.g., surveys, database searches) and sampling procedures (e.g., random selection, convenience sampling) to describe substantive areas covered in doctoral dissertations, methods used in the dissertations, and the extent to which the research is practice/intervention based. The study that is reported here makes a Canadian contribution to the understanding of doctoral education in social work.

The dissertation is the culminating step in the awarding of the PhD in almost all doctoral programs. Although programs and schools vary in the purposes of the dissertation, most would agree that the dissertation involves demonstration of a least two capacities: first, the ability to conduct independent research on an important problem in the field; second, the ability to make an original contribution to existing knowledge (Isaac, Quinlan, & Walker, 1992). As such, an in-depth understanding of social work dissertations may help the field better understand the broader topic of doctoral social work education.

The objective of this article is to describe doctoral dissertations emerging specifically from PhD programs in Canada. Findings will provide the social work profession with a sense of how the academy is "reproducing" itself, the expertise that has been developed to influence practice and policy, substantive areas that are well represented, and where there are gaps. Such an evidence base will contribute to a national dialogue about what this means for the future "stewards of the discipline" in the Canadian context.

## Research Questions

The main objective of this study is to describe the nature of doctoral social work scholarship in Canada over a 10-year period, from 2001 to 2011. There are two sets of research questions; the first set uses data across the 10-year period and provides an overall representation of the output of doctoral dissertations.

1. How many publically available dissertations are produced in Canadian Schools of Social Work?
2. What are the most commonly studied methods and topics in Canadian social work?
3. What methods are used to study the most commonly studied topics?
4. How do design features vary across research methods?

The second set of subquestions addresses comparative data within any particular year and over time, offering information about trends in social work knowledge production over the first decade of the 21st century.

5. How do research methods vary over time?
6. How does intervention vary over time?

## METHOD

This is a scoping review (Arksey & O'Malley, 2005) of publicly available dissertations. A scoping review is a form of systematic review that rapidly maps key concepts, sources, and types of evidence available in a particular area of study.

## Inclusion and Exclusion Criteria

Social work dissertations published between 2001 and 2011 at Canadian schools or faculties of social work were eligible for inclusion in the study. The 10-year inclusion window corresponds roughly to the period following the introduction of the evidence-based practice movement in social work. In addition, the timing begins 10 years after the influential 1991 Task Force on Social Work Research study in the United States, claiming a crisis in social work research (Task Force on Social Work Research, 1991) and the 2000 report on social work in Canada, *In Critical Demand* (Stephenson, Rondeau, Michaud, & Fidler, 2000). Dissertations jointly published with another discipline or dissertations published as a "special case" doctoral dissertation (from schools which may not have had a formal doctoral program at the time) were included. Dissertations written in French or English were eligible for inclusion; full-text dissertations that were not publically accessible were excluded.

## Search Strategies

An initial sample was found through the ProQuest Dissertations and Theses Database using the search terms "social work" and "Canada" and limited to doctoral dissertations. This search yielded a sample of 176 dissertations on record during the sampling period between 2001 and 2011. Second, school deans/directors (or doctoral program directors) for the 14 social work schools in Canada known to have doctoral programs in social work were contacted independently to verify the initial list of dissertations. They (or their designates) reported an additional 102 dissertations, bringing the total to 278 social work dissertations between 2001 and 2011. Only full-text dissertations were retrieved for review in our study. A total of 30 dissertations were duplicates and thus were eliminated, yielding a final sample of 248.

## Coding Procedure

A database was created using EpiData Manager 1.3.0.1, and codes were entered using the corresponding entry client program from EpiData. Variables extracted from each dissertation were defined and operationalized by our research team in two steps. First, four researchers coded the dissertations. Two of the coders were professors of social work, with experience in both quantitative and qualitative methods. The main coder was an MSW student and research assistant. A francophone MSW graduate assisted with verifying and coding some of the French dissertations. The research assistant initially coded all 248 dissertations. Questions regarding uncertain application of codes were brought to the other two senior research team members for discussion. Forty-eight dissertations that were unclear on any codes were flagged by the research assistant for additional review. The two senior team members then reviewed the flagged dissertations independently. Fifty-five single codes were in disagreement, resulting in an agreement level of 0.78. Conflicts on all the 55 codes were discussed and resolved among the research team. In the second step, the two senior research team members independently coded a random selection of 20 dissertations. The raters disagreed on two codes, yielding a final interrater agreement level of .98.

Each dissertation was coded as described by the dissertation author. Wherever possible, we did not interpret the study beyond the description by the author. For example, when an author indicated that his or her study used a phenomenological approach, we coded it as such and did not apply any appraisal criteria to ascertain whether the study met our understanding of what constituted phenomenology.

Next we describe only the variables used in this analysis. The full data set by Rothwell, Lach, and Blumenthal (2013) is available on the Dataverse Network.[2]

## Variables

### Substantive Area of Study

Each dissertation was coded to exemplify the key substantive area it addressed. The Society for Social Work Research (SSWR) topic cluster areas were used to classify each dissertation; there are 18 predefined SSWR 2014 conference topic clusters. When there was ambiguity between one substantive area and another, the "dominant" theme of the dissertation prevailed. Dissertations that could not be clearly placed into one of the SSWR categories were coded as "Other." Examples of dissertations that could not be coded into existing SSWR categories were those that focused on child custody agreements/disputes/arrangements, family and relationship issues not pertinent to work or socioeconomic status, or adoptions not related to child welfare.

### Method

Method was a categorical variable coded for all dissertations. Each dissertation was reviewed and determined to adopt one of the major method paradigms in social science: quantitative, qualitative, or mixed method. The first two categories were straightforward; any study that collected, analyzed, and combined quantitative and qualitative data was categorized as mixed methods (Creswell & Clark, 2007).

### Design

Design was a categorical variable coded based upon three categories of study design: descriptive, explanatory, and other. Those that sought only to describe phenomena, without systematically linking concepts, were coded as descriptive. Those which sought to explain phenomena via an applied causal analysis were coded as explanatory. These were typically dissertations that tested explicit hypotheses or where hypotheses were embedded in the research questions. Those that were not purely descriptive or explanatory were coded as other. For example, if some exploratory analyses were

---

[2] Data and codebook are freely available. The Dataverse Network is an open source application to publish, share, reference, extract, and analyze research data. It facilitates making data available to others and allows one to replicate other's work. Researchers, data authors, publishers, data distributors, and affiliated institutions all receive appropriate credit (http://thedata.org/).

conducted (e.g., no prior hypotheses identified and no predictive relation-ships implied by research questions), these studies were coded as other.

INTERVENTION

Intervention was coded as a dichotomous variable and therefore indicated whether the dissertation addressed an intervention. An intervention was defined as "an action undertaken by a social worker or other helping agent, usually in concert with a client or other affected party, to enhance or maintain the functioning and well-being of an individual, family, group, community, or population" (Schilling, 1997, p. 174). A dissertation was coded as exam-ining an intervention if it looked at the impact or process of an intervention (as defined by Schilling).

TYPE OF DATA

Type of data was a categorical variable that classified dissertations into ones that utilized primary, secondary, or both primary and secondary data.

# RESULTS

The first step of the analysis revealed the production of dissertations across Canadian schools/faculties of social work. Names of all the schools included in the review and results appear in Figure 1. By far, the University of Toronto has produced the most PhD graduates in the country ($n = 76$). University of Calgary has produced the second most ($n = 44$), followed by Wilfrid Laurier University ($n = 30$) and McGill University ($n = 30$). The average number of graduates per year per school was 2.48. Five schools have doctoral programs but had not yet graduated many students (i.e., fewer than five across the 10-year sampling period).

Next, using the SSWR topics, we described the most frequently studied areas of social work in Canada (see Figure 2). International topics were the most commonly studied ($n = 26$). In addition to international social work, health and disability ($n = 25$), child welfare ($n = 24$), race and ethnicity ($n = 23$), and mental health ($n = 19$) were the most studied areas. The least frequently studied topics (<5) were research design, substance abuse, and school social work. The average number of dissertations by topic was 13, with a range from 2 to 26.

Qualitative research was by far the most common method used. At 65.3% of all dissertations, the ratio of quantitative (16.9%) to qualita-tive was 1:3.9 (ratio for mixed methods [17.7%] was very similar). Further, the majority of studies were descriptive (68.5%), and most did not include a hypothesis (82.3%). Most dissertations did not include an intervention

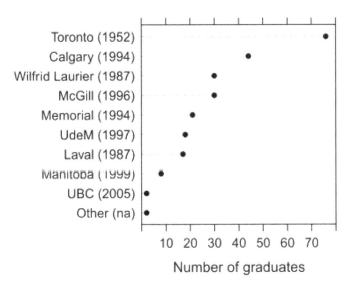

**FIGURE 1** Number of PhD graduates in social work in Canada 2001–2011. Date of first graduate appears in parentheses. "Other" includes University of Regina, Windsor University, Carleton University, York University, and McMaster University. UdeM = Université de Montréal; UBC = University of British Columbia.

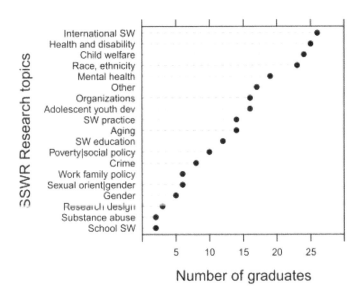

**FIGURE 2** Number of dissertations by Society for Social Work Research (SSWR) research topic 2001–2011. Topics are derived from the research categories defined by the SSWR. Examples of topics in the Other category included child custody agreements/disputes, disaster response, adoption not related to child welfare, and the subcategories under adolescent development. dev = development.

**TABLE 1** Description of Research Methods Used in Canada

| Variable | $N$ | % |
|---|---|---|
| Method: Qualitative | 162 | 65.3 |
| Quantitative | 42 | 16.9 |
| Mixed | 44 | 17.7 |
| Design: Descriptive | 170 | 68.5 |
| Explanatory | 51 | 20.6 |
| Other | 27 | 10.9 |
| Hypothesis | 44 | 17.7 |
| Intervention | 72 | 29.0 |
| Data type: Primary | 217 | 87.5 |
| Secondary | 22 | 8.9 |
| Multiple | 9 | 3.6 |

**TABLE 2** Bivariate Summary by Research Method

| Study feature | Qualitative $n = 162$ % ($n$) | Quantitative $n = 42$ % ($n$) | Mixed $n = 44$ % ($n$) |
|---|---|---|---|
| *Design* | | | |
| Descriptive | 88% (143) | 17% (7) | 45% (20) |
| Explanatory | 3% (5) | 79% (33) | 30% (13) |
| Other | 9% (14) | 5% (2) | 25% (11) |
| *Hypothesis* | 0 | 74% (31) | 30% (13) |
| *Intervention* | 24% (39) | 40% (17) | 36% (16) |
| *Data type* | | | |
| Primary | 95% (154) | 60% (25) | 86% (38) |
| Secondary | 3% (5) | 38% (16) | 2% (1) |
| Multiple | 2% (3) | 2% (1) | 11% (5) |

component (71%) and primary data collection dominated (87.5%). Results are shown in Table 1.

Of those that were coded as qualitative or mixed methods ($n = 206$), 26% were self-described as qualitative description, 22% as grounded theory, 12% as phenomenology, 10% as case studies, 5% as ethnography, and 2% narrative; 23% were not classified at all.

To understand the research methods used, we examined the bivariate relationship between method (quantitative, qualitative, mixed) and design (descriptive, explanatory, other), hypothesis driven (yes, no), intervention (yes, no), and type of data (primary, secondary, mixed). Over the entire sample, 21% ($n = 51$) of the designs were explanatory. Not surprisingly, 88% of the qualitative studies were categorized as descriptive compared to 79% of the quantitative methods that were explanatory. Regarding type of data, across method, most studies in social work used primary data (95%, 60%, 86%, respectively for qualitative, quantitative, and mixed methods; see Table 2).

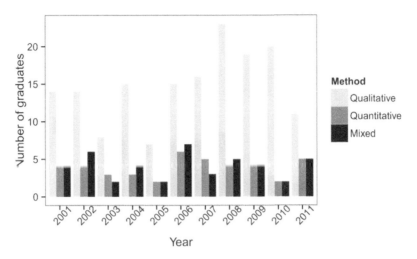

**FIGURE 3** Number of dissertations by research method over time.

## Analysis Over Time

The next part of the analysis examined trends over time; Figure 3 shows how research methods varied. Over this 10-year period, qualitative methods were consistently the most common. The ratio of qualitative to quantitative dissertations ranged from 1.4:1 in 2005 to 5.75:1 in 2008. Across time, the average number of graduates per year who conducted various dissertations was 15 qualitative, four quantitative, and four mixed. The number of graduates who conducted a quantitative thesis in any given year was never more than six.

Figure 4 shows the frequency of dissertations that examined some type of intervention as defined by Schilling (1997). We found that a majority of dissertations were not intervention based (71%). Although it was common for dissertations to not include an intervention focus, the relationship varied across time. The ratio of nonintervention studies to intervention studies ranged from lowest in 2005 (5:6) to highest in 2004 (19:3).

## DISCUSSION

Although most doctoral dissertations have been produced by eight out of 14 existing doctoral programs, six more schools have initiated doctoral pro grams since 2000. Despite this growth, there is no coordinated effort to understand the supply and demand for qualified academics to teach in schools of social work in Canada. It is therefore timely to take stock of patterns in doctoral dissertations and to reflect on their significance for social work scholarship in Canada. In this first study of its kind, we document the

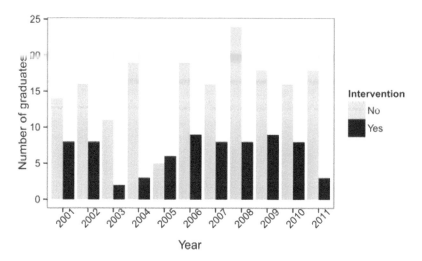

**FIGURE 4** Number of dissertations with an intervention component over time.

nature of doctoral dissertations in the country over a 10-year period. There is good reason to believe this description of social work doctoral dissertations is representative of the knowledge that is being produced in the discipline. Our results provoke several discussion points about doctoral education in social work and the nature of the profession and education in Canada.

First, there is a significant variation in the number of dissertations produced by each institution. This appears to be a function of the number of years a program has been in place and resources, reflected in the number of faculty available to supervise doctoral students. The University of Toronto has produced the greatest number of graduates. They are the longest standing doctoral program in Canada, do not deliver a BSW program (MSW and PhD only), and have one of the largest number of faculty in the country.

Compared to social work dissertations in other countries, Canadian doctoral students are more likely to employ qualitative methods (65.3%). This compares to 50% in Sweden (Dellgran & Hojer, 2001) and 40% in the United Kingdom (Scourfield & Maxwell, 2010). At 22%, qualitative research is even less common in the United States (Maynard, Vaughn, & Sarteschi, 2014). The percentage of qualitative dissertations in Canada is more similar to the rate observed in Taiwan (67%; Shek et al., 2007).

Within qualitative research, the most common methods used were qualitative description (23%), grounded theory (22%), and phenomenology (11%). These findings differed from an analysis of 75 randomly selected qualitative dissertations completed between 2008 and 2010 in U.S. schools (Gringeri et al., 2013). In that study, grounded theory was similarly used twice as often as phenomenology. However, qualitative description was not one of the categories. In our study, qualitative description, a recognized qualitative method (Sandelowski, 2000), was used to capture dissertations that used straightforward content/thematic analysis or that self-categorized as qualitative description. (An additional 26% were not classified, as they did not fit into one of the predetermined categories.) This is a significant departure from what was observed in Gringeri and colleagues' (2013) study, where only 11% were classified as "other" or "narrative" (a method not included in our study). These findings suggest that Canadian doctoral students appear to be using a broader spectrum of qualitative methods when compared to their US peers. At the same time, a significant proportion of Canadian scholars are using a more generic inductive qualitative analysis to perform descriptive research, a pattern not observed elsewhere. The heavy reliance on qualitative inquiry is problematic for the state of social work knowledge because such methods usually do not systematically build and advance our understanding of complex human and social behaviors.

The predominance of qualitative methods compels us to ask a few questions about social work doctoral education in Canada. What explains the imbalance between quantitative and qualitative dissertations? Why is the percentage of qualitative dissertations threefold higher in Canada compared to the United States? Institutional structures (e.g., the doctoral curriculum) could be a partial explanation. Whereas the relatively small number of quantitative studies does not mean that graduates aren't trained to perform a full spectrum of research, a cursory look at curriculum raises questions. Most Canadian doctoral programs require one quantitative research methods course. Consider the contrast between the University of Toronto, which mandates two quantitative and one qualitative, and McGill University, which requires just one research methods class, which may be quantitative *or* qualitative. Among schools, the University of Toronto, with the most research methods course requirements, had the highest proportion of their graduates conducting quantitative dissertations (27%). Also related to curriculum is the way research methods are taught. The goal of most graduate methods courses is for students to comprehend the concepts and theories. Comprehension is the first step. To be a competent researcher requires *mastery* of the applications of a given method. The current research course requirements of most PhD programs in Canada appear inadequate to achieve such mastery. In addition to curriculum issues, we suspect that most doctoral programs may lack the human capital necessary to teach in-depth research methods. As Figure 2 notes, there were only three Canadian graduates in 10 years whose dissertations focused on research methodology.

At the student level, another explanation for the high proportion of qualitative studies is that graduate students self-select to conduct qualitative method at an overwhelming rate compared to quantitative. This could be attributed to several factors. Previous research has documented social work students' reluctance to engage in research and anxiety about learning requisite statistics and quantitative methods (Epstein, 1987; Forte,

1995; Morgenshtern, Freymond, Agyapong, & Greeson, 2011). Based on our teaching of 1st-year doctoral students, some lack basic numeracy skills. Further many doctoral students enter the program after several years of direct social work practice where, in some settings, there is limited exposure to quantitative studies. Further, depending on the time lag and student experience in their earlier education, master's-level quantitative research methods knowledge often must be relearned in the doctoral program. This reality presents a strong start-up barrier to doctoral-level quantitative research competence. To address the disjointed nature of research methods education, social work scholars have outlined principles for establishing a continuum across the undergraduate to graduate curriculum (Fraser, Jenson, & Lewis, 1993). In addition, research on social work education has demonstrated that exposure to rigorous research and relationships with faculty are likely to have a positive impact on the attitudes of students (Morgenshtern et al., 2011). Assuming the number of doctoral dissertations being produced using qualitative methods is a reflection of the social work professorate (i.e., seven of 10), aspiring doctoral students may not have adequate exposure to high-quality quantitative social work research mentoring.

Last, graduate students frequently struggle with the perceived disconnect between the values of social work and quantitative research (Calderwood, 2012). It is common for them to perceive that quantitative research is conducted only from a positivist stance where the goal is to be entirely objective and establish absolute truth. Often such a positivist approach is equated with an oppressive research agenda that serves the status quo and further marginalizes minorities and other disadvantaged groups in society. Based on the troubling history of positivist academic research in some communities, there may well be good reason to be skeptical. In our experience, the perception among many Canadian social work students is that quantitative research is not the primary domain of the social work profession. However, this perception is anachronistic and flawed. To address the research method imbalance in Canadian doctoral social work education will require the field to move beyond these false dichotomies of the mid-20th century. The postpositivist epistemological approach to social work research that acknowledges "many ways of knowing" is a more realistic framework for how social work knowledge may be developed.

Beyond the qualitative–quantitative imbalance, our findings on design and intervention raise concern about the state of systematic inquiry for knowledge building. Consider that the vast majority (four of five studies) of social work dissertations in Canada are descriptive and that most are not intervention based. (However, the Canadian rate of 29% intervention is higher than reported in the United States, where only 13.49% of dissertations produced by doctoral students in 2006 addressed an intervention [Horton & Hawkins, 2010].) Taken together, only 21 of 248 studies were explanatory and intervention based. As found in earlier reviews of social work publications (Fraser, Taylor, Jackson, & O'Jack, 1991), we fear that the descriptive nature of social work dissertations in Canada is not generating theory to understand complex individual and social behaviors. Even among the qualitative studies ($n = 206$), most were descriptive ($n = 52$; 25%). Only 22% ($n = 46$) were grounded theory. Moreover, we are concerned that the descriptive and nonintervention nature of the scholarship has limited social impact. This trend may position social work research at the "curbside" for influencing policy and practice (Stoesz, Karger, & Carrilio, 2010). To be relevant, social work needs to address the problems confronting practitioners, administrators, policymakers, and the clients they serve. To address these problems, we require solutions beyond pure description. We recognize that intervention research is complicated and costly to design, and occurs after issues of recruitment and measurement have been adequately piloted and feasibility has been established. For these reasons, intervention research may not be the best choice for dissertations.

Moving forward, it is highly unlikely that research methods will achieve the balance called for by Shera (2003). Faculty tend to mentor and supervise students using the paradigm within which their own research is located. In this way, the reproduction of social work scholarship becomes circular and unlikely to change in the short term.

The paucity of quantitative research extends beyond dissertations in Canada. A cursory review of the 41 articles in the past seven issues of the single social work journal in the country—*Canadian Social Work Review*—revealed just two quantitative studies. This imbalance can be addressed a few ways. First, to address the possible lack of social work faculty to teach research methods, schools might hire instructors outside the discipline, from allied fields with much stronger quantitative traditions such as sociology and economics. At present, such hiring practices are observed much less frequently in Canada than in other countries. Schools also could hire faculty trained in social work from other countries where the quantitative traditions are more robust. A second action would involve systematic curriculum investments to enhance research training in general, and quantitative research training in particular. We believe that one course is not sufficient for students to learn the theoretical and conceptual framework and gain the technical expertise to conduct high-impact research. Some would argue that these skills can be learned in the student–supervisor relationship, in elective coursework, via in-service training or in the dissertation phase itself. However, we believe a structured institutional requirement embedded in the curriculum is the surest way to address the present imbalance Canadian doctoral programs could commit to requiring at least four research and statistics methods courses prior to the comprehensive exam. To master social work research then requires hands-on skill-focused training and application (Fraser et al., 1991). These quantity and quality issues require open debate and discussion.

Currently there is no institutional framework in Canada to unite PhD program directors, with or without their school or faculty deans and directors. The CASWE should embrace a leadership role in addressing the current research imbalance and capacity. Over time, institutional commitment and cultural change may slowly build the research capacity of doctoral students who will likely become the next generation of faculty. If action is not taken, we expect the status quo will be maintained and the patterns observed in this study will continue. At the same time, we recommend that CASWE also consider how building of research capacity is reflected in the quality of curricula at the BSW and MSW levels in schools of social work. Still further, there is a need for deans and directors to better understand the emerging supply-and-demand crisis with respect to preparing a sufficient number of qualified academics in Canada for the immediate future.

Turning our attention back to the topics of study, we observed a very low frequency of dissertations that specialized in substance abuse, research methods, or school social work. This has implications for practice, research, and administration of social work programs. Substance abuse and school social work are key practice areas in Canada for graduates from BSW and MSW programs (Stephenson et al., 2000). Yet we have produced few scholars who can teach them or who can produce research in these key areas of practice. A lack of expertise in research design, research methods, and measurement has similar implications for the education of social work practitioners and even more so for doctoral students.

Finally, as we move toward an era of "big data," the lack of secondary data dissertations merits discussion. In Canada, only 9% of dissertations used secondary data. Statistics Canada provides highly detailed micro data in Research Data Centres via the Canadian Research Data Network.[3] There has been a push to make this data available and accessible to researchers, yet social work appears to underutilize these resources. Secondary analysis of existing data may facilitate quicker progression through the program and allow for the development of advanced explanatory analytical techniques (Guo, 2014). We therefore would encourage doctoral programs to promote more secondary data analysis.

## Limitations

We make note of the limitations inherent in this study. The database included only published and available doctoral dissertations. It is possible that dissertations were completed but were not included in our review. Nevertheless,

---

[3] A Research Data Network is a university-based laboratory, staffed by a Statistics Canada Analyst, that offers researchers secure access to (a) confidential microdata—Statistics Canada census and surveys, plus a growing range of administrative data—and (b) fully equipped workstations, statistical software, and technical support (http://www.rdc-cdr.ca/).

we believe this study is the most comprehensive review of Canadian social work doctoral education to date. Although we took great efforts to ensure codes were used consistently, forcing codes into one category was, at times, challenging. This was particularly true for variables pertaining to topics and research design. Having said that, interrater reliability showed an acceptable level.

## Future Research

Future research should focus on more specific components of the dissertation. For example, this database lends itself to identifying theories used to guide doctoral dissertations. Critical appraisal frameworks such as the STROBE for observational designs and CONSORT for experimental designs could be used to conduct a critical appraisal of the dissertations (Equator Network, 2014). Where this study focused on design and method, more in-depth focus is needed to understand qualitative and quantitative analysis techniques. Further research also might shed light on the diverse ways in which grounded theory and phenomenology were operationalized. Replicating work in the United States (Maynard, Vaughn, Sarteschi, & Berglund, 2012), a follow-up study of the extent to which the dissertations produced in Canada appear in peer-reviewed journals, or the extent to which the researchers end up receiving tri-council funding would give us some indication of the potential "impact" of our doctoral programs. Like Oprisko, Dobbs, and DiGrazia (2013), we also are interested in understanding the relationship between doctoral education and career trajectories into the academy. Future study could also include a systematic analysis of doctoral curricula and an analysis of the trends of published research by Canadian social work faculty.

## CONCLUSION

As the number of doctoral programs increases, social work educators in Canada need to reflect on the knowledge created by and for the discipline. Although the current expansion is promising, the extent to which this phenomenon has resulted in intellectual progress is unknown. In this study we identified several issues and trends in doctoral education in Canada. The predominance of qualitative methodologies suggests that doctorates in social work are contributing to a depth of understanding related to critical social processes and problems. However, findings also raise questions about their ability to generate diverse forms of knowledge that contribute to evidence-informed policies and practices. We are concerned about the tendency for social work scholarship to be descriptive and not connected to intervention. These concerns, raised elsewhere (Lindsey & Kirk, 1992), are not unique to

Canada and speak to the creative tension in the social work profession about the centrality of research and its proper role in the academy.

## ACKNOWLEDGMENTS

We extend thanks to Nico Trocmé for constructive advice on the final draft. Josianne Lamonthe provided excellent research assistance.

## REFERENCES

Anastas, J. W., & Congress, E. P. (1999). Philosophical issues in doctoral education in social work: A survey of doctoral program directors. *Journal of Social Work Education, 35*, 143–153.

Anastas, J. W., & Kuerbis, A. N. (2009). Doctoral education in social work: What we know and what we need to know. *Social Work, 54*, 71–81. doi:10.1093/sw/54.1.71

Arksey, H., & O'Malley, L. (2005). Scoping studies: Towards a methodological framework. *International Journal of Social Research Methodology, 8*, 19–32. doi:10.1080/1364557032000119616

Brun, C. (1997). The process and implications of doing qualitative research: An analysis of 54 doctoral dissertations. *The Journal Social & Social Welfare, 24*, 95–112.

Calderwood, K. A. (2012). Teaching inferential statistics to social work students: A decision-making flow chart. *Journal of Teaching in Social Work, 32*, 133–147. doi:10.1080/08841233.2012.670065

Council of Ontario Universities. (2012). *Position paper on graduate education in Ontario* (No. 0-88799-473-3). Toronto, Canada: Council of Ontario Universities. Retrieved from http://www.cou.on.ca/publications/reports/pdfs/graduate-education-in-ontario—position-paper-(1)

Creswell, J. W., & Clark, V. L. P. (2007). *Designing and conducting mixed methods research*. Wiley Online Library. Retrieved from http://onlinelibrary.wiley.com/doi/10.1111/j.1753-6405.2007.00097.x/full

Dellgran, P., & Höjer, S. (2001). Mainstream is contextual: Swedish social work research dissertations and theses. *Social Work Research, 25*, 243–252. doi:10.1093/swr/25.4.243

Dellgran, P., & Höjer, S. (2012). The politics of social work research—Ph.D. theses in Sweden. *European Journal of Social Work, 15*, 581–597. doi:10.1080/13691457.2012.710875

Epstein, I. (1987). Pedagogy of the perturbed: Teaching research to the reluctants. *Journal of Teaching in Social Work, 1*, 71–89. doi:10.1300/J067v01n01_06

Equator Network. (2014). *Enhancing the quality and transparency of health research*. Retrieved from http://www.equator-network.org/

Forte, J. A. (1995). Teaching statistics without sadistics. *Journal of Social Work Education, 31*, 204–218.

Fraser, M., Jenson, J. M., & Lewis, R. E. (1993). Research training in social work: The continuum is not a continuum. *Journal of Social Work Education, 29*, 46–62.

Fraser, M., Taylor, M. J., Jackson, R., & O'Jack, J. (1991). Social work and science: Many ways of knowing? *Social Work Research and Abstracts, 27*, 5–15. doi:10.1093/swra/27.4.5

Gringeri, C., Barusch, A., & Cambron, C. (2013). Examining foundations of qualitative research: A review of social work dissertations, 2008–2010. *Journal of Social Work Education, 49*, 760–773.

Gripton, J. (1982). Canadian doctorates in social work: A survey report. *Canadian Journal of Social Work Education/Revue Canadienne D'éducation En Service Social, 8*(1/2), 59–73.

Guo, S. (2014). Shaping social work science: What should quantitative researchers do? *Research on Social Work Practice.* Advance online publication. doi:10.1177/1049731514527517

Horton, E. G., & Hawkins, M. (2010). A content analysis of intervention research in social work doctoral dissertations. *Journal of Evidence-Based Social Work, 7*, 377–386. doi:10.1080/15433710903344066

Isaac, P. D., Quinlan, S. V., & Walker, M. M. (1992). Faculty perceptions of the doctoral dissertation. *The Journal of Higher Education, 63*, 241–268. doi:10.2307/1982014

Lindsey, D., & Kirk, S. A. (1992). The continuing crisis in social work research: Conundrum or solvable problem? An essay review. *Journal of Social Work Education, 28*, 370–382.

Lyons, K. (2002). Researching social work: Doctoral work in the UK. *Social Work Education, 21*, 337–346. doi:10.1080/02615470220136902a

Maynard, B. R., Vaughn, M. G., & Sarteschi, C. M. (2014). The empirical status of social work dissertation research: Characteristics, trends and implications for the field. *British Journal of Social Work, 44*(2), 267–289.

Maynard, B. R., Vaughn, M. G., Sarteschi, C. M., & Berglund, A. H. (2012). Social work dissertation research: Contributing to scholarly discourse or the file drawer? *British Journal of Social Work.* Advance online publication. Retrieved from http://bjsw.oxfordjournals.org/content/early/2012/11/03/bjsw.bcs172.short

Morgenshtern, M., Freymond, N., Agyapong, S., & Greeson, C. (2011). Graduate social work students' attitudes toward research: Problems and prospects. *Journal of Teaching in Social Work, 31*, 552–568. doi:10.1080/08841233.2011.615287

Oprisko, R. L., Dobbs, K. L., & DiGrazia, J. (2013). *Placement efficiency: An alternative ranking metric for graduate schools* (SSRN Scholarly Paper No. ID 2374397). Rochester, NY: Social Science Research Network. Retrieved from http://papers.ssrn.com/abstract=2374397

Reisch, M. (2002). The future of doctoral social work education in the United States: Questions, issues, and persistent dilemmas. *Arete, 26*, 57–71.

Rothwell, D. W., Lach, L., & Blumenthal, A. (2013). *Social work doctoral scholarship in Canada (Version V2).* Cambridge, MA: Harvard Dataverse Network. Retrieved from http://hdl.handle.net/1902.1/21789

Sandelowski, M. (2000). Whatever happened to qualitative description? *Research in Nursing and Health, 23*, 334–340. doi:10.1002/1098-240X(200008)23:4<334::AID-NUR9>3.0.CO;2-G

Schilling, R. F. (1997). Developing intervention research programs in social work. *Social Work Research*, *21*, 173–180. doi:10.1093/swr/21.3.173

Scourfield, J., & Maxwell, N. (2010). Social work doctoral students in the UK: A web-based survey and search of the index to theses. *British Journal of Social Work*, *40*, 548–566. doi:10.1093/bjsw/bcn165

Shek, D. T., Lee, J. H., & Tam, S. Y. (2007). Analyses of postgraduate social work dissertations in Taiwan: Implications for social work research and education. *International Social Work*, *50*, 821–838. doi:10.1177/0020872807077915

Shera, W. (2003). Ideas in action: Doctoral social work education in Canada: History, current status and future challenges. *Social Work Education*, *22*, 603–610. doi:10.1080/0261547032000142706

Stephenson, M., Rondeau, G., Michaud, J. C., & Fidler, S. (2000). *In critical demand: Social work in Canada* (Vol. 1) (Final report prepared for the Social Work Sector Study Steering Committee). Ottawa, Canada: Canadian Association of Schools of Social Work–Association Canadienne Des Écoles de Service Social.

Stoesz, D., Karger, H. J., & Carrilio, T. E. (2010). *A dream deferred: How social work education lost its way and what can be done.* New Brunswick, NJ: Transaction.

Task Force on Social Work Research. (1991). *Building social work knowledge for effective services and policies: A plan for research development.* National Institute of Mental Health. Retrieved from http://www.socialworkpolicy.org/publications/iaswr-publications/building-social-work-knowledge-for-effective-services-and-policies-a-plan-for-research-development-a-report-of-the-task-force-on-social-work-research-november-1991.html

Yelaja, S. (1991). Doctoral social work education: A Canadian perspective. *Arete*, *16*, 63–77.

# Content and Process in a Teaching Workshop for Faculty and Doctoral Students

ELAINE S. RINFRETTE

*Department of Social Work, Edinboro University, Edinboro, Pennsylvania, USA*

ELAINE M. MACCIO

*School of Social Work, Louisiana State University, Baton Rouge, Louisiana, USA*

JAMES P. COYLE

*School of Social Work, University of Windsor, Windsor, Ontario, Canada*

KELLY F. JACKSON

*School of Social Work, Arizona State University, Phoenix, Arizona, USA*

ROBIN M. HARTINGER-SAUNDERS

*School of Social Work, Georgia State University, Atlanta, Georgia, USA*

CHRISTINE M. RINE

*Social Work Department, Plymouth State University, Plymouth, New Hampshire, USA*

LAWRENCE SHULMAN

*School of Social Work, University at Buffalo, The State University of New York, Buffalo, New York, USA*

*Teaching in higher education is often not addressed in doctoral education, even though many doctoral graduates will eventually teach. This article describes a biweekly teaching workshop, presents pitfalls and challenges that beginning instructors face, and advocates pedagogical training for doctoral students. Led by a well-known social work scholar Lawrence Shulman, the workshops were a place for participants to share their concerns and process solutions. Here, each student's scenario serves as a backdrop for Dr. Shulman's explanation of classroom content and process, for which the workshop served as a parallel process. This discussion is framed by the extant literature on preparing higher education instructors during the course of doctoral education.*

A majority of doctoral students enter academia after graduation (National Science Foundation, 2009), and as full-time faculty they will likely spend most of their time teaching (Golde & Dore, 2001). Yet most doctoral programs neglect to prepare their graduates adequately for this pedagogical responsibility (Ishiyama, Miles, & Balarezo, 2010). In their sample of 4,114 doctoral students in their 3rd year or later, Golde and Dore (2001) found that only 36.1% felt prepared by their program to teach undergraduate lecture courses, and a mere 23.3% felt prepared to teach graduate courses.

A persistent theme voiced during the teaching workshops led by one of the authors (Shulman) has been the lack of preparation and support provided for new instructors. When training was provided, it usually focused on issues such as creating a syllabus, preparing assignments, grading, lecturing, and using small-group discussions. These topics are important; however, they overlook the issues that create the greatest stress for both new and experienced instructors. In this article the workshop leader (last author) and six former doctoral student-instructors explain the rationale and structure of an ongoing, voluntary biweekly teaching workshop for full- and part-time faculty and doctoral students. The focus of the workshop was on the teaching-learning process with a special emphasis on group dynamics that occur in the classroom that may both increase and suppress student learning. We present participants' accounts of how this workshop enhanced their own teaching skills, which made for better student learning in the classroom. This workshop supports the Council on Social Work Education's (CSWE) revised 2008 Educational Policy and Accreditation Standards (CSWE, 2012). (Video recordings of workshop sessions [Shulman, n.d.] can be accessed free of charge by visiting http://socialwork.buffalo.edu/information-faculty-staff/teaching-resources/skills-dynamics-teaching-addressing-hidden-group-in-classroom.html)

## PEDAGOGICAL TRAINING FOR DOCTORAL STUDENTS

Preparing doctoral students for teaching is important for several reasons. Many graduates of social welfare doctoral programs go on to academic positions where teaching is a major component of their work (Dinerman, Feldman, & Ello, 1999; Golde & Dore, 2001; Holland, Austin, Allen-Meares, & Garvin, 1991; Meacham, 2002). In a study of position announcements in the *Chronicle of Higher Education* over a 1-year period ($N = 354$), 60% of those that itemized job responsibilities specified teaching in the department's MSW program, 53% in the BSW program, and 11% in the doctoral program (Anastas, 2006). New faculty members find themselves in institutions of higher learning that increasingly are placing emphasis on excellence in teaching, as well as scholarship and service (Valentine et al., 1998; Whicker, Kronenfeld, & Strickland, 1993).

The Group for the Advancement of Doctoral Education in Social Work Task Force on Teaching surveyed 51 social work doctoral program directors regarding how they prepare doctoral students for teaching and found that they do so in a variety of ways (Dinerman et al., 1999; Valentine et al., 1998). These include having students be graduate teaching assistants, field liaisons, or adjunct faculty; giving class presentations and guest lectures; taking a course on education; and having faculty members as mentors. Approximately one third of the programs had a teaching practicum (Knight & Lagana, 1999), whereas others responded that preparing students to teach was not a major role for doctoral social work education (Dinerman et al., 1999; Valentine et al., 1998). In fact, only 22% of doctoral program directors reported a focus on teaching in their respective programs (Anastas & Congress, 1999).

In a focus group held at an Annual Program Meeting of the Council on Social Work Education, eight new faculty members identified the need for coursework on teaching skills, styles, effectiveness, strategies, creativity, and student–teacher boundaries. These themes appear to buttress those identified in the Group for the Advancement of Doctoral Education in Social Work study (Dinerman et al., 1999; Valentine et al., 1998). New faculty members have reported spending extensive amounts of time preparing for courses and addressing concerns during the teaching process. This can delay attention to the faculty members' wishes and need to pursue their research goals, which can impact the tenure process (Boice, 1991). In addition, well-developed teaching skills allow for a sense of self-competence for the instructor and can provide a pleasurable experience in the classroom that directly benefits students (Strom-Gottfried & Dunlap, 2004), while schools of social work fulfill their goal of teaching excellence.

The social work literature, nonetheless, offers little guidance on how best to prepare doctoral students and new faculty for the important role of teacher. Absent from the discussion is a description of a reflective process, similar to the practice supervision we require of our BSW and MSW students (Sussman, Stoddart, & Gorman, 2004). This article adds to what is known by presenting such a process of reflection and the firsthand experiences of the facilitator and participants.

## RATIONALE FOR THE TEACHING WORKSHOP

New instructors, at a time they feel most vulnerable, often are afraid to raise their concerns with colleagues. Untenured faculty uniformly express a worry that if they confront an issue in class, particularly one related to a subject such as race, gender, or sexual orientation, and do not handle it well, they will face grievances or accusations of bias. If they confront problematic students, they may receive negative comments on their teaching evaluations and hurt their chances of obtaining tenure. What new instructors often miss is that much of their own substantial understanding about practice can inform them as they take on this new role. Although the class is an educational enterprise, and not a therapeutic encounter, much of what they have learned about practice can be adapted to the context of teaching.

The reality of a *parallel process* argues for providing preparation and support for new faculty. For example, when an instructor is teaching about empathy and confrontation in a practice class, but demonstrates little of either in the teaching role, students are witnessing the disjuncture between what is said and what is done. The expression "more is caught than taught" aptly describes how students are influenced by what they feel and perceive in the classroom. The proposed workshop uses reflection and group process skills learned in practice to increase new instructors' awareness of teacher–student interactions and improve their teaching efficacy.

## TEACHING WORKSHOP

This workshop was developed at the SUNY Buffalo School of Social Work and was structured as an informal and voluntary opportunity for doctoral student instructors and new faculty to meet biweekly and discuss teaching issues. The workshop was open to faculty and doctoral student instructors to join at any time, sessions were held on an ongoing basis, and participants were welcome to attend regularly or less consistently, as their need warranted and schedule allowed. Discussion topics roughly followed the phases of work, focusing on the preparation (tuning in), beginning (contracting), middle (work), and ending and transition phases of the semester (Shulman, 2011). Early examples focused on first classes issues (engaging students, overcoming apathy, dealing with challenges to authority), later sessions focused on classroom management, and the last sessions of the workshop dealt with grading and ending and transition issues.

At the start of each session, participants were asked to share their concerns and examples from their current or past classes, and to use "memory work" to re-create the process of the class in question during the workshop. Thus, the seminar consisted of presentations, examples, discussion, and mutual aid among participants. The group leader facilitated discussions about classroom dynamics and potential responses. An important element of the workshop was to create a culture where participants felt safe taking risks and comfortable sharing honest feedback in a supportive manner. The leader encouraged everyone to learn from mistakes, go back and try a different intervention, and then make "more sophisticated mistakes." It was important for participants to understand that this is a lifelong professional process as they learn from their experiences, their colleagues, and their students how to continually improve their teaching skills. In this way, the workshop modeled the integration of process and content.

The balance of the article explores specific examples discussed in the workshop. All contributors and coauthors have written their examples in the first person and in their own style, adhering to an agreed-upon structure with the following elements: problem description, impact on the instructor, workshop discussion, intervention effort, outcome of the intervention, and next steps. After each student's contribution, a "commentary" has been added from the perspective of the workshop leader.

## Engaging Students in First Classes Under Difficult Circumstances

WORKSHOP PARTICIPANT

Once my first course was assigned, I was concerned about everything from how to properly translate goals and objectives into assignments to how to construct a grading rubric. I was especially concerned about setting the right tone on the first day. Although my knowledge of the material was solid, my comfort level in teaching was shaky.

On my first day I felt prepared, excited, and optimistic. I was met with what I perceived to be 16 very disinterested and passive social work students. Our first 2 hour and 45 minute session together began with the customary first class activities: a getting-to-know-each-other exercise, review of the syllabus, overview of the format in which course material would be presented, and an introduction to how the ecological perspective would frame the material.

I soon learned that many of the students already knew each other quite well from other classes; this led to my "get to know you" exercise being poorly received and beneficial only to me. What I thought was a clear syllabus was in fact very unclear to many of the students who voiced concerns. Reviewing the format of the class led to a discussion of "How come we have to do presentations and role-play in every class?" Finally, my transition into the use of the ecological perspective was met with "Why do we have to know the macro stuff? We are not in the community concentration!" This entire discourse took place in a room without windows that was upwards of 70 degrees and that had residual unpleasant odors from a previous class group. Student comments about our less than ideal environment were interspersed throughout the discussion. I left this first class feeling utterly defeated.

I was pleased that our teaching workshop was going to take place a day later. Once in our workshop session, I was relieved to find that others faced similar issues with their first class. Before I had a chance to raise my concerns, we were already in a discussion initiated by other participants that also addressed my issues. This provided me with a safe environment to jump in with my dilemmas.

The workshop leader addressed these concerns by reframing the teaching environment into something that we were all able to relate to: group work with clients. Once he laid out the similarities of these two seemingly different groups and presented examples of group work techniques to apply to the classroom, it started to make sense. My "self-talk" immediately changed to "I know how to do this; I have done this for years."

As the semester unfolded, what I initially saw as student disinterest and passivity turned out to be an expression of other concerns: fatigue, busy schedules, too many responsibilities, feeling overwhelmed at the start of a new semester, and anxiety about upcoming graduation and subsequent career changes that accompany this transition. Although I did not have the ability to affect these issues, I understood that I had to acknowledge these very real student concerns in order to move past the negative impact they had on our first class session together.

For our second class, I followed a plan developed through insight gained at our workshop by addressing criticisms and issues from our first session. I discussed the benefits of collegial support from one's fellow classmates for both academic and personal concerns. I reviewed the syllabus to clarify assignments and addressed the importance of presentations and role-play, as they directly relate to real practice situations. In a similar manner, I gave a case example illustrating how the ecological perspective is not just for community concentration social workers. Finally, the elephant in the room was the room itself. Openly acknowledging our hot, smelly room was enough for it to become a nonissue. In fact, this *problem* became the running joke that bound us together throughout the semester.

These early lessons provided me with the foundation of my teaching style, which continues to be under construction as I learn from each new experience in the classroom. In my new role of instructor, the greatest impact the teaching workshop had on me was in its ability to instill self-confidence. Not only did I feel more competent in handling classroom problems, I also knew the workshop would be there for me when I needed guidance. The only thing that remained the same was that we still had a classroom with no windows, but it did not seem to matter.

## WORKSHOP LEADER'S COMMENTARY

One of the most powerful impacts of the teaching workshop was the relief that came from the mutual aid process called the "all-in-the-same-boat" phenomenon (Shulman, 2011). This changes the dynamics in the participant's class from one that is personal to one that is universal. The workshop presentation content that framed the class term as having a beginning, middle, and ending also allowed for an understanding of the students' concerns and behavior as related to the dynamics of beginnings (in the academic context) and with being an authority figure. This remained an important theme throughout the workshop: Individual and group behavior always has meaning, often indirectly expressed, and our job is to try to understand it.

## Facilitating Learning in Challenging Courses

### WORKSHOP PARTICIPANT

It was my first class teaching research methods, and I could tell by the look on my students' faces that they did not share my enthusiasm for research. As a new professor teaching master's-level social work students, I contemplated how I could help students become more engaged in learning research course material. It was as a participant in the teaching workshop here during my doctoral studies that I discovered the answers to this important question.

### LEARNING TO "TUNE IN"

During the sharing stage of one particular workshop session, I described my dilemma to the participants and was prompted by the facilitator to reflect on my experiences as a social work student taking research courses. Looking back, I realized, similar to the students in my class, I too dreaded research courses, finding them boring and disconnected from social work. By reflecting on my past experiences as a student in a research course, I was able to empathize with the discouragement students felt in my own classroom. The act of "tuning in" out loud with my workshop colleagues helped me recognize how important it was in my research courses to facilitate active learning and draw the important connection between research and practice.

The notion of "tuning in" to students and instructing "with" them instead of "to" them became the central theme for that particular workshop session discussion. Over the course of the hour, participants shared personal strategies and techniques that they used in their own courses to help break up the monotony of the lecture and actively engage the students in learning course content. With their support, I was encouraged to incorporate multiple experiential activities to enhance student learning. These activities included small-group exercises, debate forums, student presentations, and visual media.

One activity that I used that students found particularly helpful and relevant to their work in the field was a "show-and-tell" exercise. This assignment required students to locate a research article or advertisement in a journal or popular magazine, provide a brief description of the research, critique it, and present the implications for practice to the class. For instance, one student brought in an article from *Good Housekeeping* advertising the benefits of a specific antidepressant on treating adolescent depression. This particular student did a great job critiquing the research methods of the study and reported how the antidepressant was only minimally effective with a small

71

homogeneous sample of adolescents. The student's presentation prompted an engaging class discussion on the growing "movement to medicate" in mental health and how this may negatively impact the clients we serve. The experiential activity engaged students in the process of learning because it allowed them to see a more direct connection between social work practice and research, and because it was much less boring than my lectures.

The teaching workshop taught me how important it is for instructors to tune in to their students as they would with their clients in practice. By relating to the anxiety and apprehension some students feel in challenging courses like research, I was able to deploy experiential activities to help transform my classroom into a more engaging and active learning environment. I will continue to incorporate what I learned in the workshop about the process of teaching throughout my academic career.

WORKSHOP LEADER'S COMMENTARY

In addition to designing a more interesting and engaging course structure, the instructor in this case also included a discussion with students in the first class about previous experiences with research, statistics, and their inability to see a connection to practice. As is often the case, under the surface of the initial resistance ("Why do we have to take research?") is a fear of the difficulty they anticipate with research methods in general and statistics in particular. Once this underlying issue surfaces, it tends to lose power, which allows the instructor to explore steps to address the concern.

## Dealing With the First Class: Challenges to the Instructor's Authority

WORKSHOP PARTICIPANT

As a new BSW program instructor, I struggled with the issue of students challenging my authority as a professor. However, I lacked confidence on two levels. First, I was still a student. I did not have my PhD prior to my first teaching experience. I thought students might perceive this as a lack of expertise, despite my 13 years of practice experience. Second, I never taught a college-level course. I was experienced in providing presentations and trainings to other professionals in the community, and I was quite comfortable doing so. However, nothing prepared me for the challenges of the college classroom.

The initial issue that arose during the first class was whether students could call me by my first name. The students stated, "It makes professors more approachable." I agreed to the students' request, hoping it would help us to engage as a group. I had little insight into the problems this would create. A second issue was my physical appearance and age. Students said I looked too young to be a professor. I became somewhat anxious, anticipating the challenges I might encounter based on a stereotypical image of what a professor is supposed to look like (whatever that is). I struggled with how to remain true to who I was, yet be credible and gain the respect of my students as a university professor. The third undercurrent was related to course expectations. I was a bit discouraged when my students did not demonstrate my passion for the social work profession or for high-quality work.

Prior to the workshop, I attempted to avoid the awkwardness of the first class by routinely using it as a "freebie." Essentially, I avoided addressing the process that was taking place in the classroom. The second class, I started right in with my lecture, leaving little opportunity for discussion. As a result, there was a fragmented, disconnected feeling for the remainder of the semester.

At first, I felt uncomfortable bringing up my issues in the teaching workshop. I did not know all of the members. I knew that some of the participants taught courses before, and that was somewhat intimidating. However, as the workshop unfolded, I realized I was not alone. Other participants struggled with some of the exact same issues. I sat around the table listening intently, waiting for the perfect moment to bring up my concerns. I remember likening it to sitting in class, trying to think of something brilliant to say. When that moment never came, I decided I would need to take a risk if I wanted to grow as an educator. As a group, we generated a number of tangible ideas and suggestions to implement. The different skill levels and the willingness of participants to open up allowed for a rich discussion around how to address my uneasiness in the classroom during those first few classes.

Throughout the seminar, it became clear that the workshop leader was actually modeling how to deal with these issues through his interaction with the group. He masterfully orchestrated a safe environment conducive to rich dialogue among members. He paid attention to the verbal and nonverbal cues as they were unfolding and addressed them immediately. Over time, it became clear that our group's dynamics paralleled those in the classroom. If we choose not to respond to classroom behaviors (direct and indirect), we are essentially giving permission for them to occur. In the end, we were setting the stage for ongoing problems that could potentially influence the learning process for others.

I returned to the classroom ready to implement the suggestions gleaned from the seminar. When students made comments about my age, I engaged them in a brief conversation about what I believed the real issue may be—their concern that I may not be qualified to teach them the material they were there to learn. They seemed responsive to dialogue. The less focused I was on the issue, the less focused they were. Additionally, now I have changed the way I handle first classes. I no longer let classes out early. I prepared a structured first class agenda with activities that demonstrated my expectations of students in the course. I spent a great deal of time on activities that would create a safe environment to maximize learning. I kept students the entire class time, sending a message about the importance of the course material. In addition, I made it routine to structure the physical setting of the classroom in order to invite dialogue (as opposed to lecturing at them).

The seminar helped me define my role as an educator. I learned to be comfortable articulating when course expectations were non-negotiable. I now work exceptionally hard to understand what my students' behaviors and cues are telling me before I move on to further discussions. Addressing what is happening in the classroom seems to send a clear message to students that we are all active participants in the learning process. It appears to eliminate (or at least significantly reduce) distractions that impede learning for others.

WORKSHOP LEADER'S COMMENTARY

This entry is marked by the complete honesty of the instructor, who expresses very clearly the sense of anxiety that new faculty often feel but will not admit. It is her ability to be in touch with these feelings, to understand where they originate, and then to take steps to address them directly that can lead to significant growth. The instructor here understands that it is important to reach for the real questions under the question "How old are you?" The students want to know if the instructor will be able to teach a competent course. By responding directly to the indirect cues, the instructor models the exact behavior that will be needed when the young, unmarried worker is asked by his or her first client, "And how many kids do you have?" It is also important that the instructor presents a professional role and demeanor, thus modeling for the students what will be expected of them as professional social work practitioners.

Responding to a Student Raising Personal Mental Health Issues

WORKSHOP PARTICIPANT

I was teaching a class on mental health interventions when I was asked about the impact of childhood trauma on current mental health symptoms. I stressed the importance of asking questions about history, and then I explained that certain patterns of symptoms could suggest past abuse. When I cautioned the students about the possibility that assessment questions could trigger intense feelings, a student responded by saying that she was able to discuss her own past experiences with her therapist without any such feelings being triggered.

I was not sure how to respond to the student. I did not want to discuss her personal therapy or her past life experiences in class. I also did not want to say that she should not discuss such personal experiences in class, and wondered whether the comment was the type of reaction that I had been explaining. If I acknowledged the student's statement without commenting on it, I could be modeling therapeutic avoidance for all the students. However, discussing her personal therapy would be inappropriate in class. Instead, I suggested that there were many different experiences in counseling sessions. Then I changed the subject by presenting a different example from my own clinical experience.

I presented this event during the workshop, because I was not satisfied with my response. I specifically wondered how to better address the student's statement, and in general how to respond to the possibility that class discussions could trigger personal responses among students. The group suggested that I acknowledge that some classroom discussions were likely to parallel student experiences, and then lead a group discussion to explore how students' feelings could get triggered in class and also in field. In addition, this discussion could explore the students' concerns and uncertainty about helping a person with background trauma. This approach would generalize the discussion, rather than focusing on an individual student's personal experiences.

I was able to use the workshop suggestion in my next class. I referred to the previous class discussion of trauma and invited students to discuss their concerns about recognizing these effects and about making some mistake that would exacerbate the client's symptoms. The students discussed many concerns, including how their own feelings and life experiences may interfere with providing effective therapy.

This class discussion was a positive learning experience for them and for me. While I could easily respond to a person's feelings in my clinical work, I lacked experience in interpreting individual comments in the role of an instructor and in the context of a class. This experience also increased my confidence about responding to student comments about personal experiences while respecting the importance of boundaries.

WORKSHOP LEADER'S COMMENTARY

This instructor's experience provided an opportunity for an important workshop discussion on the issue of the educational contract and the role of the instructor. It is not uncommon, especially for an experienced practitioner who is new to teaching, to suffer from "functional diffusion" in which lack of clarity about the purpose of the educational encounter and the role of the instructor may lead to inappropriate personal discussions in a classroom. By not opening up discussion of a student's personal experiences—either the disclosed early abuse or the current experience in therapy—the instructor appropriately "guards" the educational contract and protects the student. Other students need to see that they also will be protected if they disclose personal information and that the instructor will not turn the class into a therapeutic encounter.

## What to Do When You Don't Know the Answer

WORKSHOP PARTICIPANT

Even though research tells us that instructors do not have to be perfect geniuses in the classroom, I can still feel uncomfortable when faced with a content-related question I cannot answer. One theme in the workshop that came through to me, and seemed to run through all of the sessions, is that of being human. Our workshop facilitator modeled for those present that there is no greater skill, and perhaps no greater gift, than to be human with our students. To illustrate his point, the facilitator gave a number of examples, some embarrassing, in which his honesty and spontaneity was the best way to connect with a class.

What I took away from the workshop was how to forgive myself for not being perfect in the classroom and how to model for students, as the facilitator modeled for us, that making a mistake is okay, that it doesn't diminish who we are as people or professionals, and that we really can address our mistakes and live to see another day. All of this can be operationalized by the following five strategies I learned from the workshop that are helpful when in doubt in the classroom: (1) Do not ignore errors. "Students expect expertise but they are also realistic—and perceptive" (Magnan, 1990, p. 1). If you make a mistake, say so. Correct it and move on. (2) Do not pretend to know the answer. "If you can't answer a question, admit it, then find out" (Magnan, 1990, p. 1). (3) Do not gloss over a student's question. (4) Do not deny your mistake. Never have I earned students' respect more than when I owned up to a mistake. I now consider mistakes an opportunity to demonstrate humility and responsibility-taking to my students. (5) Do not waste the students' time. Be honest. Instructors expect students to take ownership when not prepared. Do the same to show them how it is done. "Admit that you're unprepared and ask the class how the time can best be spent" (McKeachie, 1994, p. 219). Also, make sure you are prepared in the future—make this occasion the exception.

WORKSHOP LEADER'S COMMENTARY

This example of a willingness to be honest and not needing to have all the answers was written by a former PhD student with extensive and successful teaching experience; however, this confidence was acquired over time. The irony is that just when you need to be most honest about what you don't know, as you start your teaching career, is the time when it is most difficult to do so. In teaching, as in practice, we only think we can hide our real feelings from those with whom we work. In reality, students are very sensitive receivers of our signals and can identify incongruity between what we feel and what we say. Successful practice and teaching involves finding a way to integrate the two.

## Dealing With a Negative Instructor Evaluation

WORKSHOP PARTICIPANT

The first class I taught in the MSW program while a doctoral student was usually taught by a very popular and knowledgeable faculty member, but the teaching assignment was changed a few weeks prior to the beginning of the semester. Students had signed up for the course thinking they would be taught by the experienced faculty member.

The school routinely asks students to complete an anonymous course evaluation prior to midterm. The results are provided to the instructor. The comments that I received were mixed. While there were several positive ones, I focused on those that were negative. Bringing this up in the seminar took a lot of courage. I had been attending this workshop for over a year and had respect for the leader, the process, and my colleagues. So I believed I had little to lose and a lot to gain. I revealed my mortifying evaluation and my response to it.

The workshop leader focused on the purpose of the midterm evaluation and how to use it constructively in class. It was common practice that evaluation results were not shared with students by the instructor. The facilitator suggested that I take the results of the evaluation back to the students and discuss positive and negative responses. In addition, he suggested that I comment on the negative areas that I could change, address the areas that I could not change, but also ask for student input on how to make them more palatable and to identify areas where *students* would need to take more responsibility for what was occurring in class.

While this was frightening to consider, I was very excited about doing it. I liked this idea for several reasons. It was novel. I had never been in a class where this was done, and I thought it would show respect for the students' efforts in filling out the evaluation. I liked it because it made me feel less responsible for "fixing" everything. I could explain why certain aspects of the class were the way they were, take responsibility for my shortcomings and discuss my plans to improve, and also hold the students responsible for their part in the learning process.

I followed through with the plan at the beginning of the next class. The students seemed surprised that I was doing this but were very responsive. They offered options and strongly suggested that I be myself and not try to emulate the faculty member who was supposed to have taught the course.

They were very positive about what I had to offer the class based on my clinical experience and knowledge of the didactic material.

The intervention provided me some relief and went better than I expected. I think the students felt they knew me better and appreciated my candor. In addition, I believe the students felt respected and felt that they were part of the process of improving the learning environment of the class. My final evaluation was quite different. Comments made by students were very positive and encouraging of my continued efforts to find my own teaching style.

## WORKSHOP LEADER'S COMMENTARY

This was a crucial area for discussion in the workshop. By understanding the midterm questionnaire as a "formative" evaluation, one designed to impact the rest of the semester, it becomes obvious, although scary, to take the next step of talking with the students about the results. The instructor's comment that this seemed to be rare is on target, and yet she also understands that this is a way to demonstrate courage, openness to feedback, and respect for the students. In this way, students are asked to become partners in the educational enterprise, and one of their important roles is to provide honest feedback to the instructor.

## DISCUSSION

Here, six doctoral student instructors shared their teaching stories, experiences not unlike those of other new instructors who have reported similar struggles and concerns (Orr, Hall, & Hulse-Killacky, 2008). Approaches, such as the ones described here, have demonstrated success in preparing doctoral students for the teacher role. Burton, Bamberry, and Harris-Boundy (2005) found that introducing student-instructors to their assigned courses, providing them with teaching strategies and techniques, and having them learn from successful experienced teachers improved teaching efficacy. The present workshop provided participants with these experiences and went further by encouraging personal reflection, peer support, and feedback.

The workshop also modeled a reflective process for evaluating classroom interactions and helped participants view problematic classroom experiences in terms of group process rather than as personal failings or inadequate skills. Applying this model to future teaching experiences can promote ongoing discussions in which colleagues share stories of both successful and challenging teaching experiences. Potentially, this process not only improves individual teaching skills but also promotes an ongoing collegial commitment to learning that can support teaching skills across a faculty, and thereby improve student learning.

## Implications for Higher Education

The participant-authors advocate the practice of providing a reflective workshop for new instructors as a place to share process and content of their teaching experiences. In a parallel process, the facilitator modeled honesty, humility, and humanity, all the while adding to the conversation based on his years of teaching, practice, and leadership experience. Other supervisory models exist, such as weekly, biweekly, or monthly one-on-one or group supervision sessions, but these meetings usually cover several teaching responsibilities, of which classroom content and process is but a part (Davis & Kring, 2001; Levin, 2008; Orr et al., 2008).

Preparing Future Faculty (PFF) is a national effort to groom doctoral students for a career in academia. PFF (n.d.) prepares doctoral students for faculty responsibilities, provides them with mentors, and joins various academic departments and types of higher learning institutions into small collaborative clusters. Several colleges and universities offer such a program to their students, and some provide empirical support as to its effectiveness (e.g., Gerdeman, Russell, & Eikey, 2007). Many institutions implement the program using a courselike approach, having students participate in a single- or multiple-semester seminar. However, not all implementations offer a reflective workshop for new classroom teachers (Gerdeman et al., 2007), which we argue is a valuable component. Moreover, PFF has been criticized by faculty who perceive the program's overemphasis on teaching support, at the expense of research mentorship, which may compromise doctoral students' learning opportunities and the university's research standing (Jones, Davis, & Price, 2004). However, Gale and Golde (2004) argued that good teachers make good researchers. We point out that, unlike a formal program such as PFF, a biweekly teaching workshop does not impede doctoral students' involvement in other learning opportunities, but rather is one crucial part of a larger effort to prepare such students for the responsibilities that await them.

## WORKSHOP LEADER'S CONCLUDING THOUGHTS

One of the most enjoyable aspects of leading a teaching workshop is to watch new instructors become excited by the subject of teaching. At first tentatively—until reassured that making mistakes and learning from them is part of the process—they begin to look at their own role in the teaching–learning process. As they gain new insights, take risks in the workshop, and then take risks in their classrooms, their confidence grows. They develop the ability to tolerate ambiguity and stay open to new learning. They grow in their understanding that learning to be an effective instructor is a professional, lifelong process and that they can draw upon colleagues, mentors, and their own students for help along the way.

# REFERENCES

Anastas, J. W. (2006). Employment opportunities in social work education: A study of jobs for doctoral graduates. *Journal of Social Work Education, 42*, 195–209. doi:10.5175/JSWE.2006.200400426

Anastas, J. W., & Congress, E. P. (1999). Philosophical issues in doctoral education in social work: A survey of doctoral program directors. *Journal of Social Work Education, 35*, 143–154.

Boice, R. (1991). Quick starters: Faculty who succeed. In M. Thean & J. Franklin (Eds.), *Effective practices for improving teaching* (pp. 111–121). San Francisco, CA: Jossey-Bass.

Burton, J. P., Bamberry, N.-J., & Harris-Boundy, J. (2005). Developing personal teaching efficacy in new teachers in university settings. *Academy of Management Learning & Education, 4*, 160–173. doi:10.5465/AMLE.2005.17268563

CSWE Commission on Accreditation. (2012). *2008 EPAS handbook.* Retrieved from http://www.cswe.org/File.aspx?id=64764

Davis, S. F., & Kring, J. P. (2001). A model for training and evaluating graduate teaching assistants. *College Student Journal, 35*, 45–51.

Dinerman, M., Feldman, P., & Ello, L. (1999). Preparing practitioners for the professoriate. *Journal of Teaching in Social Work, 18*, 23–32. doi:10.1300/J067v18n01_05

Gale, R., & Golde, C. M. (2004). Doctoral education and the scholarship of teaching and learning. *Peer Review, 6*(3), 8–12.

Gerdeman, R. D., Russell, A. A., & Eikey, R. A. (2007). A course to prepare future faculty in chemistry: Perspectives from former participants. *Journal of Chemical Education, 84*, 285–291. doi:10.1021/ed084p285

Golde, C. M., & Dore, T. M. (2001). *At cross purposes: What the experiences of today's doctoral students reveal about doctoral education.* Retrieved from http://www.phd-survey.org/report%20final.pdf

Holland, T., Austin, D., Allen-Meares, P., & Garvin, C. (1991). An octennium of doctorates: Trends in characteristics of doctoral students in social work and other fields during 1981-1988. *Arete, 16*, 1–11.

Ishiyama, J., Miles, T., & Balarezo, C. (2010). Teaching the next generation of teaching professors: A comparative study of Ph.D. programs in political science. *PS: Political Science and Politics, 43*, 515–522. doi:10.1017/S1049096510000752

Jones, A. L., Davis, S. N., & Price, J. (2004). Preparing future faculty: A new approach at North Carolina State University. *Teaching Sociology, 32*, 264–275. doi:10.1177/0092055X0403200302

Knight, C., & Lagana, M. (1999). The use of a teaching practicum for doctoral students in social work. *Journal of Teaching in Social Work, 18*, 13–22. doi:10.1300/J067v18n01_04

Levin, E. (2008). Career preparation for doctoral students: The University of Kansas history department. *New Directions for Teaching and Learning, 113*, 83–97. doi:10.1002/tl.310

Magnan, R. (1990). *147 practical tips for teaching professors.* Madison, WI: Atwood.

McKeachie, W. J. (1994). *Teaching tips: Strategies, research, and theory for college and university teachers* (9th ed.). Lexington, MA: D. C. Heath.

Meacham, J. (2002). Our doctoral programs are failing our undergraduate students. *Liberal Education, 88*, 22–28.

National Science Foundation. (2009). *Table 43. Employment sector of doctorate recipients with definite postgraduation U.S. employment commitments, by sex, citizenship, and race/ethnicity: Selected years, 1989-2009*. Retrieved from http://www.nsf.gov/statistics/nsf11306/appendix/pdf/tab43.pdf

Orr, J. J., Hall, S. F., & Hulse-Killacky, D. (2008). A model for collaborative teaching teams in counselor education. *Counselor Education & Supervision, 47*, 146–163. doi:10.1002/j.1556-6978.2008.tb00046.x

Preparing Future Faculty. (n.d.). *The Preparing Future Faculty program*. Retrieved from http://www.preparing-faculty.org/

Shulman, L. (n.d.). *The skills and dynamics of teaching: Addressing the hidden group in the classroom*. Retrieved from the University at Buffalo School of Social Work website: http://socialwork.buffalo.edu/resources/resource-center/product.html?id=6

Shulman, L. (2011). *The skills of helping individuals, families, groups and communities* (7th ed.). Belmont, CA: Cengage.

Strom-Gottfried, K., & Dunlap, K. (2004). Talking about teaching: Curricula for improving instructors' classroom performance. *Journal of Teaching in Social Work, 24*, 65–78. doi:10.1300/J067v24n03_05

Sussman, T., Stoddart, K., & Gorman, E. (2004). Reconciling the congruent and contrasting roles of social work teacher, student and practitioner: An experiential account of three doctoral students. *Journal of Teaching in Social Work, 24*, 161–179. doi:10.1300/J067v24n01_10

Valentine, D., Edwards, S., Gohagan, D., Huff, M., Pereira, A., & Wilson, P. (1998). Preparing social work doctoral students for teaching: Report of a survey. *Journal of Social Work Education, 34*, 273–282.

Whicker, M. L., Kronenfeld, J. J., & Strickland, R. A. (1993). *Getting tenure*. Thousand Oaks, CA: Sage.

# Preparing PhD-Level Clinical Social Work Practitioners for the 21st Century

JOAN BERZOFF and JAMES DRISKO

*School for Social Work, Smith College, Northampton, Massachusetts, USA*

*Social work doctoral programs are not adequately preparing students to educate future clinical practitioners. Social work is predominantly a practice profession. Social work's PhD programs must continue the education of excellent researchers while also educating for excellence in practice, teaching, field liaison, and the supervision of practice. Nevertheless, The Group for the Advancement of Doctoral Education in Social Work (GADE) and the social work profession have heavily emphasized the education of researchers over the past 20 years but have neglected the practice needs of the profession at a time when client diversity has increased and available social supports have decreased. This article examines shifts in academic priorities, in funding, in hiring practices, and in accreditation standards that have reduced the quality and support for clinical practice education in social work. We also explore the much-reduced research expectations of social work's emerging DSW programs. We recommend continued recognition and strong support for PhD education in social work, with a clear and extensive clinical practice component, as well as explicit attention to the education of PhD-level practitioner/researchers as leaders in social work education and in practice research. Affirmation by GADE and by the social work profession and its professional organizations is needed for educating leaders in clinical social work.*

Doctoral educators are responsible for preparing the future stewards of the social work profession. The Group for the Advancement of Doctoral Education in Social Work (GADE), in its 1992 and 2003 *Guidelines for Quality in Education in Social Work Doctoral Programs*, stated that "social work doctoral programs have as their primary purpose the production of scholars/educators who disseminate knowledge concerning social welfare problems and professional practice" (GADE, 2003, p. 1). In this article we examine the professional practice portion of this mission, addressing how and why we believe practice preparation and practice experience are essential components of PhD education.

We contend that social work doctoral graduates who seek to teach and do research on practice need to have substantial direct engagement in advanced practice before and during their doctoral programs (Belcher, Pecukonis, & Knight, 2011) in order to train and acculturate future BSW and MSW students into professional practice. We also feel that those who educate future practitioners need prior experience working in social agencies. Educators of practice and practice theory must be able to understand and convey a core body of knowledge, values, and skills based in environmental and sociocultural contexts, grounded in psychological theories, and linked with evidence-based research knowledge. Doctoral graduates who will teach practice, therefore, must be socialized in their doctoral programs to use empirical evidence, apply critical thinking, and engage with issues of social diversity and economic justice. Further, they must be able to use themselves consciously and flexibly in order to teach how to address a wide range of psychosocial problems and intervene with diverse client populations. Doctoral graduates above all need expertise in *doing* practice. Such experience will enable them to be both skilled and credible social work educators and role models for future practitioners, field liaisons, and practicum instructors/supervisors responsible for student socialization into the profession. PhD graduates who take leadership in practice also need to be able to frame, conceptualize, and guide practice research in a manner consistent with social work's person-in-environment perspective.

## CONTEXT OF THE PROBLEM: SOCIAL WORK IS A PRACTICE PROFESSION

According to United States Bureau of Labor Statistics (2010–2011) data, 89% of social workers in the United States work in direct practice. That is, 570,000 of the 640,000 social workers in America are employed as practitioners. The Bureau's statistics may include some "social workers" who lack professional education, but Groshong (2009) also confirmed that 96% of 310,000 state licensed social workers engage in direct practice. "Practice is our purpose," said New York City National Association of Social Workers

(NASW) former Chapter President Rose Starr, who also stated that "the profession's survival requires that we not lose our essential value to those we serve" (Starr, 2007, p. 2). Indeed, social work has always been, and remains a predominantly practice-based profession. Bogo (2010) noted that "the purpose of social work education is the education of competent social work practitioners" (p. 55). Clearly, students primarily come to BSW and MSW programs to become practitioners (Howard, Allen-Meares, & Ruffolo, 2007). Yet many authors, including Johnson and Munch (2010), Goldstein (2007), and Simpson, Williams, and Segall (2007) have argued persuasively that social work doctoral education is not adequately preparing social work scholars to teach the students who will become the majority of our profession.

## The Academy Focuses on Funding and Research

Despite calls for greater attention to education for direct practice, PhD programs have shifted markedly in the past 15 years toward educating the "star researcher" rather than preparing the future clinical practitioner/researcher (Mendenhall, 2007; Stoesz, Karger, & Carrilio, 2010). Murray and Aymer (2009) stated that there is a tension between the pressures on academic institutions and faculty to engage in grant-funded research, on one hand, and the information and leadership needs of the direct practice professions, on the other.

In a national survey, Barsky, Green, and Ayayo (2014) found that many BSW and MSW programs expressed a strong interest in hiring new faculty with practice experience. However, there is no disagreement that PhD-level social workers must be able to undertake research to inform the profession. Nonetheless, we argue that PhD programs in social work may be abdicating their responsibility as stewards of the profession in favor of stewarding only an academic discipline. Balanced attention to the need *both* to maintain excellence in research and to promote excellence in practice should be the focus of social work doctoral education.

Belcher et al. (2011) asserted that the emphasis on grant-funded research in social work doctoral education has begun to corporatize the academy. This corporatization has led to competition for limited funds that largely come from biomedical sources, which tend to exclude social workers or give them low priority. They asserted that social work's person-in-environment perspective is often minimized (or omitted) and that both teaching and practice are devalued in the education of PhD-trained social workers. Belcher et al. further maintained that the current funding of social work schools increasingly relies on federally funded grants, so "research and scholarship are shaped by the federal bureaucracy but not the needs of students, clients and the profession as a whole" (p. 201). Further, the value base of the social work profession may not necessarily be consonant with the funding priorities of the federal government. The emphasis on funded research also has reshaped faculty priorities. One impact has been the replacement of social work faculty with non-social-work hires such as those with degrees in psychology, marriage and family therapy, public health, economics, and political science.

## Increase of Faculty Without Social Work Degrees

In the effort to enhance social work's research capacity, social work education has moved away from hiring social workers. Howard and Garland (2011, p. 195) compared social work programs that were "top ranked" by *U.S. News and World Report* with similar programs in other professions. They found that a range of 51% to 86% of social work faculty held MSW degrees. They also found that between 42% and 80% of faculty held doctoral degrees in social work or social welfare. In comparison, Howard and Garland discovered that most faculty members of law, medical, dental, and nursing schools held doctorates in these professions, whereas substantial proportions of the five top-ranked social work faculties did not hold graduate MSW or PhD degrees in social work or social welfare (p. 199). We think that this apparent trend undermines professional socialization and the application of social work's core person-in-environment paradigm.

## Rapid Increase in Use of Adjunct Faculty to Teach Practice and Theory

There presently would appear to be not enough PhD credentialed social work educators to teach practice (Zastrow & Bremner, 2004). There are currently (in 2014) 233 accredited MSW programs and 500 accredited BSW programs, more than a fourfold increase since 1970. This expansion has created a need for more PhD-level educators than are graduated annually (Schilling, Morrish, & Liu, 2008). Relatively few social workers pursue doctorates; for example, only 308 degrees were awarded during the 2009–2010 academic year (CSWE, 2011). As Anastas and Kuerbis (2009) poignantly observed, "Although in some fields there seems to be an oversupply of doctoral graduates, the concern in social work is that we have too few graduates to meet current faculty needs" (p. 71). In turn, program administrators are increasingly contracting practice courses out to adjunct faculty who have no influence over the curriculum (NASW, 2011) and frequently no PhD degree. As a result, many new faculty members are being hired (inexpensively) under annual contracts as adjuncts, or on nontenured clinical faculty lines.

CSWE President Darla Coffey (personal communication, April 5, 2013) reported that, according to Council on Social Work Education (CSWE) statistics, more than half of faculty positions in CSWE accredited programs are now held by adjuncts. Moreover, McMurtry and McClelland (1997) documented a threefold increase in the use of adjunct faculty. Fagan-Wilen,

Springer, Ambrosino, and White (2006) also noted that the use of adjuncts produces a substantial cost savings for academic institutions that frees up full-time tenure-track faculty to conduct funded research. Pearlman (2013) argued that social work education's increasingly heavy reliance on adjunct faculty poses a particular ethical challenge for the profession because they are paid much less and generally carry heavy teaching and advising loads. Whereas adjuncts, in part, compensate for the inadequate supply of PhD-educated practice instructors, they are far less involved with the institutional life of academic institutions and programs (McMurtry & McClelland, 1997), and they frequently are unfamiliar with the current research literature and its implications for practice (Klein, Weisman, & Smith, 1996).

In effect, a two-tiered system has developed in social work education in which the more powerful tenured faculty are research oriented and the non-tenured clinical and adjunct faculty are more practice oriented. This trend may reshape the nature of social work education permanently, promoting a permanent split between research and practice that will not optimally serve the needs of most students who wish to engage in research-informed practice.

## Reduced Qualifications for Practice Teaching

The Education and Policy Accreditation Standards of CSWE (2008) have reduced the requirement for teaching practice in accredited programs to just 2 years' post-BSW practice experience for practice teachers and field advisors. (The prior accreditation standard required 2 years of MSW-level practice experience for these educational roles.) This reduced standard has created some serious concern among practitioners and educators (Goldstein, 2007; Johnson & Munch, 2010). Those who are teaching practice may have less experience than do their students and therefore may not always be appropriate models of skilled practitioners. Within social work faculties, there are few researchers/practitioners who can fully conceptualize assessment and practice, understand the challenges of professional uses of self, serve as practitioner role models, and conceptualize contemporary practice issues. There also are too few researchers/practitioners who can fully conceptualize real-world practice processes and outcomes to guide quality research (Valentine et al., 1998). This emerging reality compromises the quality of professional education accredited programs can offer to their students.

## Enhancing Research Presence; Reducing Practice Infrastructure

During the last 25 years, social work has undertaken a sustained, well-planned effort to increase its research capacity and access to external grant funding (Biegel, 2008). Indeed, social workers have been very effective in this endeavor (Fong, 2011). NASW (2011) underscored that PhD-level "social workers in academia are often 'faculty researchers,' involved in teaching and advising undergraduate and graduate students," as well as "researching and publishing on subjects that inform and advance the profession" (p. 1). Paradoxically, however, these efforts have reduced the number of faculty who can do and teach practice—the educators who will prepare our next generation of practitioners, supervisors, and field instructors. Many researchers are neither familiar with contemporary direct clinical practice nor rewarded for doing it (Dubois, 2012; Goldstein, 2007). This trend is eroding the kind and quality of practice education so sorely needed to face the complexity of contemporary practice (Johnson & Munch, 2010). In a time of decreased resources for clients and greater acuity of social and psychological problems (Donner, 1996), social work education appears to be deemphasizing the quality of training for our profession. This drives many MSWs to seek further postgraduate training in order to be able to practice effectively. Moreover, graduates often attend training institutes run by other disciplines and run the risk of losing their identification with the profession of social work (Goldstein, 2007; Johnson & Munch, 2010).

We thus assert that doctoral education needs to maintain its historical role in preparing future educators to take leadership in field education (Power & Bogo, 2003). In the current practice world, there are serious constraints on interns, supervisors, and field advisors (Bocage, Homonoff, & Riley, 1995; Noble & Irwin, 2009). Supervision in agencies has been eroded by external funding constraints, demands for greater productivity, risk-management issues (Gelman & Wardell, 1988), higher workloads, more students in the field with disabilities (Cole & Cain, 1996), greater exposure to violence and trauma (Donner, 1996), and managed care (Raskin & Blome, 1998). All of these influences result in less time for reflection, assessment, and ongoing treatment planning (Homonoff, 2008). Further, there is less attention to the social work student's self-knowledge (Everett, Miehls, DuBois, & Garran, 2011; Marziali & Alexander, 1991) and to intercultural competence—despite the greater diversity of contemporary client populations (Bogo, 1993). These pressures impinge upon the quality of supervision and field instruction. Academics who have had advanced training in supervision and field advising therefore must strengthen and support field instruction in contemporary practice and research. They need to be prepared to teach about evidence-based practice (Gitterman & Knight, 2013), assessment and intervention skills, and the use of theory in practice (Homonoff, 2008). Noble and Irwin (2009) wrote,

> It is beholden upon both scholars and practitioners to explore the way current knowledge about supervision can respond in a creative and relevant way to the challenges identified. We suggest that a critical lens needs to be used to review supervision theory and practice as a matter of urgency. (p. 356)

We concur that supervision and field advising are key parts of BSW and MSW education that warrant PhD-level conceptualizations of practice and research. Doctoral programs need to produce scholars who are educated to guide the practice and research parts of the social work profession as they do in other health and mental health professions.

Agencies also are alarmed by the lack of clinical preparation of social work students. Recently the Boston Area Hospital Administrators group, representing the social work leadership from 10 major teaching hospitals—five in the Harvard system—contacted Smith College School for Social Work's Director of Field Education because they no longer consider most recent MSW students from many Boston programs to be adequately trained to serve patients in medical settings. They noted that if the trend toward poor preparation for practice in social work education continues, they will train Master in Family Therapy students and will no longer train social workers at all. Such concerns as well have implications for interdisciplinary work with medical and nursing professionals from whom many academic social work researchers also receive funding (Belcher et al., 2011).

Furthermore, without researchers/practitioners on full-time faculties, intellectual leadership in contemporary practice is diminished. "Not only are academicians gate-keepers for the profession, they also shape practice through the selection of content to be taught and the articulation of objectives for their programs" (Shore, 1991, p. 233).

## GADE'S POSITION ON THE ROLE OF DOCTORAL EDUCATION

Since the 1970s, GADE consistently has endorsed three different models of doctoral education in social work. All three appear in the 1996 and 2003 GADE *PhD Program Quality Guidelines*. The first is the traditional academic PhD model "which places primary emphasis on . . . training for scholarship and pursuit of professional knowledge through scientific research" (Thomas, as cited in Shore, 1991, p. 232). The second model is the practice-oriented doctorate, designed to enhance practice skills and, at the same time, provide stimulus "to use a scholarly and analytic approach to practice" (Thomas, as cited in Shore, 1991, p. 232). Sometime around 2008, this was known as the Doctorate in Social Work (DSW) model because it generally is the course of study currently in use at these programs. The DSW includes less extensive research coursework and less demanding efforts to produce research than does the traditional PhD model. In DSW programs, mastery of theory, development of writing skills, and the application of existing research to practice are emphasized (NASW, 2013). It appears, however, that no current DSW program mandates a practice internship component.

Thomas's third model is the researcher/practitioner model (as cited in Shore, 1991, p. 232). It emphasizes education for *both* advanced practice functions *and* contributions to knowledge-based scientific research. It includes the same attention to education for research and scholarship as does the traditional PhD model but also includes education for advanced practice. PhD programs employing the researcher/practitioner paradigm may, or may not, include internship components. However, programs that educate for practice solely through classroom study may appear little different from the traditional PhD or DSW model.

Shore (1991) asserted that the emphasis of doctoral education "should be on improving practice within its social context" (p. 231). She noted that a GADE committee in fact suggested that "doctoral programs may relate to practice through the use of internships" (p. 233). Thomas and GADE both argued that "students placed in social agencies may provide a stimulus to practitioners to examine their practice more carefully or to consider the developing knowledge base of social work" (p. 233). This requires *both* education about research *and* education about practice. We concur, and view PhD field internships as vital and in vivo ways to engage doctoral students in advanced practice by exposing them to contemporary treatment methods with diverse clients, and in providing new laboratories for research. When such researcher/practitioner PhD students bring the university into the community, and the community into the university, more sophisticated conceptualizations about research and evaluation are likely to emerge.

A PhD in social work must educate for excellence in research skills but also may educate for excellence in conceptualizing, executing, and teaching practice. Unlike the DSW, PhD graduates must be knowledgeable and skilled researchers. In the terminology of CSWE's (2008) Education and Policy Accreditation Standards, master's level students *use*, but do not *produce*, research knowledge. Hence, it is imperative to have PhD-level social workers, with a mastery of practice, shaping our practice research agenda.

## THE DSW: SOMEWHAT STRONG ON PRACTICE, WEAK ON RESEARCH

Practice doctorates, created in part as a solution to the lack of clinically experienced instructors with doctoral-level credentials, offer less emphasis on research than do PhD programs but generally provide more emphasis on theories of practice through classroom study. This distinctly different emphasis raises the question of whether the practice doctorate is a form of advanced continuing education or an authentic doctoral course of study.

Anastas and Videka (2012) reviewed online materials for contemporary social work DSW programs (as of February 2012) and identified several differences between DSW and PhD programs. These include (a) more practice content, (b) less research content than found in PhD programs, (c) a lack of oral comprehensive/qualifying exams, and (d) lower dissertation expectations. The DSW degree dissertation requirements usually focus on the design of a research project, but not its completion, and do not mandate an empirical and nonempirical paper for publication or a scholarly portfolio. It should be noted that many DSW programs are new and evolving, and two new online DSW programs are now advertised, and a third is in development. (None of these new programs was included in the Anastas and Videka study.)

A small working group of the CSWE Leadership Forum prepared a preliminary report on the DSW degree (Edwards & Rittner, n.d.). The report's recommendations were quite broad. The report argued for an advanced practice degree, with several potential practice specialties or concentrations. (No practice requirements were stated.) In addition, the report also recommended modest research requirements. Indeed, the word *scholarship* was used more often than *research* in the document. The report also suggested "that faculty have a strong scholarly record in examining and disseminating scholarship on practice related topics [and] that at least one member of the faculty assigned to this program hold a current advanced practice license (e.g. LCSW or LICSW) if the program is clinical in focus" (p. 9). The suggested level for faculty involvement in practice, therefore, is relatively modest, and no specific research qualifications were mentioned for DSW faculty. One might wonder how a comparable suggestion—that at least one faculty member hold a research PhD degree at a research intensive university—might be viewed.

It is noteworthy that Levin (1991), writing in favor of a clinical doctorate in social work 24 years ago, emphasized research as a key part of a practice doctorate. He stated that a practice doctorate in social work "should be an in-depth clinical experience, including theory and practice that also includes a significant research component, and is under the auspices of the profession" (p. 236). We agree that *both* research and practice are vital parts of all doctoral-level education in social work. Nevertheless, attention to practice content in social work PhD programs appears to have declined in inverse relation to the increased attention given to research content and skills. Mendenhall (2007) noted that clinical practitioners who enter research-focused PhD programs in social work shift roles, contexts, and expectations with the message that they need new skill sets. Johnson and Munch (2010) argued that the role of practice should not be secondary to research but co-equal and that weakening practice content and practice requirements for social work educators benefits neither students nor the profession.

## STEWARDS OF THE PROFESSION, OR JUST OF THE DISCIPLINE?

Anastas (2012) opined that a key issue is whether doctoral education in the professions should be dedicated solely to preparing "stewards of the discipline" or also should address practice and service delivery. The GADE (2003) *PhD Program Quality Guidelines* notes that serving as stewards involves much more than research and knowledge development. Social work has the mandate to provide ethically guided and legally sanctioned services to the public. Every state in the United States has social work licensing requirements, but few doctoral programs are preparing teachers who are able to help their students become licensed in the field, especially at the advanced practice level.

The larger "enterprise" of social work includes practice, service delivery, policy, and social change. Both GADE (2003, p. 1) and Tucker (2003) defined social work as a (a) practice activity, (b) discipline, and (c) research tradition. Stewards of the social work profession therefore must address all three areas, including direct practice.

Although Shore (1991)—who served as the chair of GADE—did not personally endorse a practice-only doctorate (i.e., DSW), she did support *both* the researcher-practitioner model and the traditional model of PhD education in social work. She noted—and we concur—that a PhD in social work *has* to emphasize research, but PhD education can *also* emphasize practice. This is fully analogous to PhDs in psychology, nursing, and education, which are also service professions. We believe both PhD models should continue to be actively supported by GADE. Sadly, we find that such support is not fully clear in GADE's (2013) *PhD Program Quality Guidelines.*

## Research and Practice: The Researcher/Practitioner Model

The rise of the evidence-based practice (EBP) movement has added significantly to the research knowledge and skills required of social work practitioners. Contemporary definitions of EBP include four components: (a) the current clinical circumstances of the client, (b) the best relevant research evidence, (c) the client's values and preferences, and (d) the clinical expertise of the professional clinician (Rubin, 2008). To understand and apply EBP in practice, to contribute to its knowledge base, and to critically analyze EBP research requires PhD-level practice knowledge, skills, and experience (Gitterman & Knight, 2013). The kinds of quality standards and methods applied in the respected international and multidisciplinary Cochrane Collaboration and Campbell Collaboration systematic reviews are well beyond what is taught and mastered at the MSW level. Because these standards detail the highest quality outcome research, social work practitioners need to be familiar with them. Still, *doing* practice informed by the EBP model also requires clinical expertise and great skill in getting to know clients. PhD-level education in research, and involvement in producing research, is vital to such mastery. Also required for teachers of EBP is the PhD-level integration of research and practice, as both practice and research expertise are needed to comprehend and teach EBP.

In addition to understanding these systematic reviews, two other areas of research have particular relevance to social work practice. The first is empirical research on the role of relationship as a causal factor in therapeutic change. Considerable new work in psychology by Norcross and Lambert (2011) and by Castonguay and Beutler (2006), with participation by Linehan and Prochaska, provides an empirical research base for the importance of relationship to therapeutic change. Castonguay and Beutler (2006) identify both common and unique relationship factors that impact practice outcomes. Their work shows that techniques alone are not the sole factor of practice effectiveness and outcomes. Prochaska, DiClemente, and Norcross's (1992) "stages of change" model has been applied in substance abuse and mental health treatment to understand and to accommodate wide variation in client readiness to participate in change. In social work, Marsh, Angell, Andrews, and Curry (2012) noted great variation in outcomes based on the quality of client–provider relationships. They also argued for much better conceptualization of the sources of change in social work services in child welfare, substance abuse, and mental health. As a case in point, PhD-level social workers need to understand such research and be able to apply it to their own practice, research, and teaching.

The second body of practice research is the common factors approach. Recent studies by Norcross and Lambert (2011, 2012) indicate that about 40% of variance in client outcomes remains unexplained. Of the other 60% of explained variance in outcome, they assign 30% to the "client's contribution," 12% to the impact of the therapeutic relationship, 8% to the impact of specific therapeutic techniques, 7% to individual therapist characteristics and 3% to other factors (pp. 11–14). Note carefully that just 8% of variable in outcomes is assigned to specific treatment models. How specific techniques—the focus of systematic review research—intersect with variation in client capacities and resources, and with the skills of specific providers, warrants more research and much closer inspection (Cameron & Keenan, 2012). These results suggest that social work education at all levels needs to pay closer attention to educating skilled, differential, and selective practitioners.

## A VIEW FROM THE PRACTICE WORLD

For at least the last two decades, field educators have lamented the erosion of supervisors who are competent to train students due primarily to their own lack of theoretical grounding (Bucky, Marques, Daly, Alley, & Karp, 2010; Dubois, 2012; Saltzburg, Greene, & Drew, 2010). As a result, master's students are learning increasingly how research informs practice but are not instructed on how practice informs research. When research and practice are split, they often are disconnected from reality (Johnson & Munch, 2010).

Whereas students in MSW programs may be learning techniques of psychological treatment (such as mindfulness-based practice or CBT) and how to practice from manualized protocols, they are not learning how to conceptualize their practice from multiple theoretical perspectives, or how to choose among related interventions (Goldstein, 2007). Frequently, students are not being adequately taught how to optimally engage, make, and maintain clinical relationships, or how to understand the complex biopsychosocial histories that their clients present in order to intervene at individual, family, group, organizational, or community levels (Marziali & Alexander, 1991). They often are neither learning how to critique and modify their practice theories and interventions for those most at risk nor learning about how the complexity of human diversity intersects with psychological and biological theories (Berzoff, Flanagan, & Hertz, 2011; Homonoff, 2008; Noble & Irwin, 2009). In addition, many are no longer learning the value of theoretically grounded psychosocial practice that places human development in the context of powerful environmental influences (Berzoff, 2011; Goldstein, 2007; Mailick, 1991). Furthermore, students in MSW programs are not learning about differential uses of self, about their clients' effects on them, or their effects on their clients, and the difficult dynamics that occur between the two (Berzoff, 2011; Bucky et al., 2010; Goldstein, 2007; Schamess, 2012). Moreover, many are not learning about trauma, attachment, and neurobiology—despite these being well grounded in research-informed and evidence-based practice.

Content on practice at the doctoral level has declined in the past 40 years. In 1982, Orcutt and Mills found that 63% of doctoral programs offered practice courses and opportunities. Shore (1991) stated that by 1991, practice content and internship opportunities had declined markedly and only 28% of programs were offering practice internships. Groshong (2009) lamented the loss of attention to practice and practice theory in social work education, which she sees as undermining the professions' efforts to maintain and enhance state licensure. Changes in curriculum content have included less attention to developing and sustaining relationships, and to a range of practice-related theories (Goldstein, 2007). This often leads students to seek continuing education or DSWs to try to compensate for what was missing in their MSW programs (Johnson & Munch, 2010).

## THE SUPERVISOR'S PERSPECTIVE

Supervision has also been a neglected domain in doctoral education. Within 2 to 3 years of graduation, graduate students generally go on to supervise, often without having learned the skills of using case-based methods or having had the experience of using process recordings. Both of these can help their MSW interns to learn about clinical relationships through examining microinteractive clinical processes (Urdang, 1991, 1999). Increasingly, neither supervisors nor students are examining process recordings to try to decipher how relationships shape human behavior within the social environment (Nye, 2012).

Masters field placements are service apprenticeships. The role of the field instructor is to help the student integrate theories with practice; develop skills; confront ethical dilemmas; understand cultural, racial, and gendered complexities; examine personal struggles; learn deliberate uses of self; and intervene with a sense of purpose and goals (Dubois, 2012). Our content analysis of the last 2 years of *The Clinical Supervisor* journal reveals that the most important ingredients to supervision were (a) attention to use of self, (b) "responsiveness"—that good and attuned supervision aids good practice, (c) and reflexivity, which is developed only in close supervision. In current agency-based practice, however, supervisors face greater expectations for productivity, administrative documentation, and short-term crisis-oriented work in high-risk settings (Bucky et al., 2010). Further, Bucky et al. (2010) found concerns about the ability of supervisors to stay focused, meet time constraints, address professional and differential use of self, and challenge the supervisee effectively. They also question the commitment of supervisors to the supervisory alliance.

Practitioners and supervisors are increasingly obligated by funders to use a very restricted list of payer-approved treatments that often are very different from those identified in the Cochrane Library (http://www.the cochranelibrary.com/view/0/index.html) or in the Campbell Collaboration (http://www.campbellcollaboration.org/lib/) of Systematic Reviews. These treatments are not always delivered in a manner remotely consistent with evidence-based practice. This requires great expertise in assessment and treatment planning. Treatment planning, as part of evidence-based practice, must be done collaboratively with the client. Thus supervisors must be trained to help their students establish relationships in which they can conduct this process interactively.

Supervisors also need training to understand that there are empirically based models of relationship (Castonguay & Beutler, 2006) that provide an evidence-based grounding for a number of core practice skills. PhD-level social workers need to be able to help supervisors and students identify theoretical models that are likely to be a best fit with diverse client's values, social environments, and preferences, integrated with research-informed evidence.

Supervisors should also be able to help students take risks, make errors, and formulate responses to difficult and complex situations. Field instruction should be a collaborative process of making sense of process recordings, responding to impasses in clinical work, and acting with intention (Nye, 2012). Supervision should facilitate insight and change in the practitioner and help new practitioners tolerate uncertainty (Schamess, 2012).

Still, supervisors need training by PhD-level social workers to be nimble with conceptualizing clinical data, integrating theory and practice, helping students navigate ambiguity, and acting according to the best clinical judgment and current research (Bettman, Thompson, Padykula, & Berzoff, 2009). Who is preparing these supervisors for these complex tasks, especially in a practice world governed by empiricism and payers? In the typical social work PhD program, there is one course on teaching but none to prepare supervisors to socialize and acculturate students to the profession.

## CONCLUSION

We believe that social work must educate a pool of PhD-credentialed faculty with advanced practice experience, combined with strong research skills, who can provide MSW students the knowledge, values, skills, and research base for clinical practice. There must be ample social work faculty to serve as effective practice teachers and role models. These faculty members must be able to link theory to practice and to use their practice experience in teaching so that their MSW students can do the same (Knight, 2001). Anastas and Videka (2012) have reminded us that social work education needs to socialize MSW students toward the enterprise of the entire profession, not just the discipline, and that PhD-level academics need to become fully qualified to do so. This has been GADE's position for four decades. We believe that this position must be maintained by GADE and affirmed by the social work profession.

We think that doctoral students must have the capacity to appreciate and to critique practice as well as to build knowledge about practice with socially diverse clients. This must be coupled with the capacity to both use and produce research about practice. We also feel that all doctoral programs must resist the trend toward objectification and reductionism that is at odds with the need for treatment modalities that are biopsychosocial in nature and appropriate for work with neglected and traumatized populations. Manualized treatments often are overly generalized to cover most social work problems and populations (Singer & Greeno, 2013; Stegall & Nangle, 2005). This fact can become problematic if students are not learning how to conceptualize their work and critique it, to exercise clinical skills in relationships, and to develop a flexible and client-centered use of self when making differentiated biopsychosocial assessments and treatment plans. Such clinical expertise is essential to evidence-based practice. Further, we hold that PhD graduates must take leadership in teaching practice, and in supervision and advising, in order to help students meet the core competencies articulated by CSWE. Emphasizing the dignity and worth of the individual, emphasizing service, underscoring the importance of relationships, and focusing on the ways in which psychological theories do (and do not) address those who are most marginalized all are essential responsibilities of academic social work practitioners.

## AREAS FOR FURTHER DISCUSSION

This article examined trends in PhD-level education in social work over the past 30 years. We believe it has documented a continuing reduction in emphasis on social work practice education and the consequences this gradual decline has had on preparing an adequate work force for the academy. The reduction in practice education at the PhD level also impacts the quality of supervision and field advising offered to students. Hence, we support an expanded emphasis on practice-focused education in our profession's PhD programs.

Several key issues deserve further scholarship and discussion. Research-focused PhD programs have developed, in part, to meet a latent goal of providing an income stream for educational institutions that is not tuition based. This research-based income stream has supported doctoral students in research assistant roles and has offered them valuable research training. How to fund and expand practice training, which does not have such explicit sources of external funding support, is one key issue to be addressed. Educational intuitions will need to develop business models that provide support for the full range of need in both research and practice.

The curriculum of PhD programs in clinical social work also warrants ongoing review and continued development. Existing clinical PhD programs within academic institutions offer useful paradigms. The range of clinical social work theories, models, populations, and services further suggests that PhD programs with varied objectives should be created to meet new and emerging hiring and service needs. Although such programs will vary in program and emphasis due to specific institutional mission and goals, the role and focus of clinical practice education at the PhD level deserve further scholarship and discussion in support of fully addressing the hiring needs of social work programs at all levels, improving practice research, and optimally serving social work clients. As social work's knowledge base expands, as the demands on practitioners become increasingly complex, and as scholars become more removed from practice, we encourage the academy to meet its responsibility to educate PhD-level practitioners and scholars.

## REFERENCES

Anastas, J. (2012). *Doctoral education in social work*. New York, NY: Oxford University Press.

Anastas, J., & Kuerbis, A. (2009). Doctoral education in social work: What we know and what we need to know. *Social Work, 54*, 71–81. doi:10.1093/sw/54.1.71

Anastas, J., & Videka, L. (2012). Does social work need a practice doctorate? *Clinical Social Work Journal*, *40*, 268–276. doi:10.1007/s10615-012-0392-3

Barsky, A., Green, D., & Ayayo, M. (2014). Hiring priorities for BSW/MSW programs in the United States: Informing doctoral programs about current needs. *Journal of Social Work*, *14*, 62–82. doi:10.1177/1468017313476772

Belcher, J., Pecukonis, E., & Knight, C. (2011). Where have all the teachers gone? The selling out of social work education. *Journal of Teaching in Social Work*, *31*, 195–209.

Berzoff, J. (2011). *Falling through the cracks: Psychodynamic practice with vulnerable and at risk clients*. New York, NY: Columbia University Press

Berzoff, J., Flanagan, L., & Hertz, P. (2011). *Inside out and outside in: Psychodynamic theory and practice in multicultural contexts*. Lanham, MD: Roman and Littlefield.

Bettman, J., Thompson, K., Padykula, N., & Berzoff, J. (2009). Innovations in doctoral education: Distance education methodology applied. *Journal of Teaching in Social Work*, *29*, 291–312. doi:10.1080/08841230903018397

Biegel, D. (2008). Social work education: Research. In T. Mizrahi & L. Davis (Eds.), *Encyclopedia of social work* (Vol. IV, 20th ed., pp. 130–133). New York, NY: Oxford University Press.

Bocage, M., Homonoff, E., & Riley, P. (1995). Measuring the impact of the current state and national fiscal crises on human service agencies and social work training. *Social Work*, *40*, 701–705.

Bogo, M. (1993). The student–field instructor relationship: The critical factor in field education. *The Clinical Supervisor*, *11*(2), 23–36. doi:10.1300/J001v11n02_03

Bogo, M. (2010). *Achieving competence in social work through field education*. Toronto, Canada: University of Toronto Press.

Bucky, S., Marques, S., Daly, J., Alley, J., & Karp, A. (2010). Supervision characteristics related to the supervisory working alliance as rated by doctoral-level supervisees. *The Clinical Supervisor*, *29*, 149–163. doi:10.1080/07325223.2010.519270

Cameron, M., & Keenan, E. K. (2012). *The common factors model for generalist practice*. New York, NY: Pearson.

Castonguay, L., & Beutler, L. (Eds.). (2006). *Principles of therapeutic change that work*. New York, NY: Oxford University Press.

Cole, B., & Cain, M. (1996). Students with disabilities: A proactive approach to accommodation. *Journal of Social Work Education*, *32*, 339–349.

Council on Social Work Education. (2008). *Educational policy and accreditation standards*. Alexandria, VA: Author.

Council on Social Work Education. (2011). *2010 statistics on social work education in the United States*. Alexandria, VA: Author.

Donner, S. (1996). Field work crisis: Dilemmas, dangers and opportunities. *Smith College Studies in Social Work*, *66*, 317–331. doi:10.1080/00377319609517469

Dubois, C. (2012). Introduction. *Smith College Studies in Social Work*, *82*, 113–115.

Edwards, R., & Rittner, B. (n.d.). *The doctorate in social work (DSW) degree: Emergence of a new practice doctorate* (Report of the Task Force on the DSW Degree convened by the CSWE Social Work Leadership Forum). Retrieved from http://www.cswe.org/File.aspx?id=59954

Everett, J., Miehls, D., DuBois, C., & Garran, A. M. (2011). The developmental model of supervision as reflected in the experiences of field supervisors and graduate students. *Journal of Teaching in Social Work, 31,* 250–264.

Fagan-Wilen, R., Springer, D. W., Ambrosino, B., & White, B. (2006). The support of adjunct faculty: An academic imperative. *Social Work Education, 25,* 39–51. doi:10.1080/02615470500477870

Fong, R. (2011, May). *Framing education for a science of social work: Missions, curricu- 660 lum and doctoral training.* Paper presented at the Shaping a Science of Social Work Conference, Los Angeles, CA.

Group for the Advancement of Doctoral Education in Social Work (GADE). (1992). *Guidelines for quality in social work doctoral programs.* Retrieved from http://www.gadephd.org

Group for the Advancement of Doctoral Education in Social Work (GADE). (2003). *Guidelines for quality in social work doctoral programs (revised).* Retrieved from http://www.gadephd.org

Group for the Advancement of Doctoral Education in Social Work (GADE). (2013). *PhD program quality guidelines.* Retrieved from http://gadephd.org/Portals/0/docs/GADE%20quality%20guidelines%20approved%204%2006%202013%20%282%29.pdf

Gelman, S., & Wardell, P. (1988). Who's responsible? The field liability dilemma. *Journal of Social Work Education, 24,* 70–78.

Gitterman, A., & Knight, C. (2013). Evidence-guided practice: Integrating the science and art of social work. *Families in Society: The Journal of Contemporary Social Services, 94,* 70–78. doi:10.1606/1044-3894.4282

Goldstein, E. (2007). Social work education and clinical learning: Yesterday, today and tomorrow. *Clinical Social Work Journal, 35,* 15–23. doi:10.1007/s10615-006-0067-z

Groshong, L. (2009). *Clinical social work practice and regulation: An overview.* Lanham, MD: University Press of America.

Homonoff, E. (2008). The heart of social work: Best practitioners rise to challenges in field instruction. *The Clinical Supervisor, 27,* 135–169. doi:10.1080/07325220802490828

Howard, M., Allen-Meares, P., & Ruffolo, M. (2007). Teaching evidence-based practice: Strategic and pedagogical recommendations for schools of social work. *Research on Social Work Practice, 17,* 561–568. doi:10.1177/1049/31507300191

Howard, M., & Garland, E. (2011). Our best schools of social work: How good are they? *Social Work Research, 35,* 195–201. doi:10.1093/swr/35.4.195

Johnson, Y., & Munch, S. (2010). Faculty with practice experience: The new dinosaurs in the social work academy? *Journal of Social Work Education, 46,* 57–66. doi:10.5175/JSWE.2010.200800050

Klein, W., Weisman, D., & Smith, T. (1996). The use of adjunct faculty: An exploratory study of eight social work programs. *Journal of Social Work Education, 32,* 253–263.

Knight, C. (2001). The process of field instruction: BSW and MSW students' views of effective field supervision. *Journal of Social Work Education, 37,* 357–379.

Levin, A. (1991). Is there a role for clinical doctoral education: Yes! *Journal of Social Work Education, 27,* 235–238.

Mailick, M. (1991). Reassessing assessment in clinical social work practice. *Smith College Studies in Social Work*, *62*, 3–19. doi:10.1080/00377319109516696

Marsh, J., Angell, B., Andrews, C., & Curry, A. (2012). Client-provider relationship and treatment outcome: A systematic review of substance abuse, child welfare, and mental health services research. *Journal of the Society for Social Work and Research*, *3*, 233–267.

Marziali, E., & Alexander, L. (1991). The power of the therapeutic relationship. *American Journal of Orthopsychiatry*, *61*, 383–391. doi:10.1037/h0079268

McMurtry, S., & McClelland, R. (1997). Trends in student–faculty ratios and the use of non-tenure-track faculty in MSW programs. *Journal of Social Work Education*, *33*, 293–306.

Mendenhall, A. (2007). Switching hats. *Journal of Teaching in Social Work*, *27*, 273–290. doi:10.1300/J067v27n03_17

Murray, J., & Aymer, C. (2009). The apparent conflict between commitment to the development of the profession and the imperatives of the academy. *Social Work Education*, *28*, 81–95. doi:10.1080/02615470802109908

National Association of Social Workers. (2011). *Furthering your social work education: Obtaining a doctorate*. Washington, DC: Author. Retrieved from http://careers.socialworkers.org/documents/Furthering%20your%20social%20work%20education.pdf

National Association of Social Workers. (2013, September 23–24). *Advanced practice doctorate programs examined. NASW Social Work Policy Institute symposium*. Task Force meeting. Reported in the November 2013 *NASW News*.

Noble, C., & Irwin, J. (2009). Social work supervision: An exploration of the current challenges in a rapidly changing social, economic and political environment. *Journal of Social Work*, *9*, 345–358. doi:10.1177/1468017309334848

Norcross, J., & Lambert, M. (2011). Evidence-based therapy relationships. In J. Norcross (Ed.), *Psychotherapy relationships that work* (pp. 3–21). New York, NY: Oxford University Press.

Norcross, J., & Lambert, M. (2012). Evidence-based therapy relationships. Retrieved from the Substance Abuse and Mental Health Services Administration's National Registry of Evidence-Based Programs and Practices: http://www.nrepp.samhsa.gov/Norcross.aspx

Nye, C. (2012). Introduction to theoretical perspectives. *Smith College Studies in Social Work*, *82*, 122–123. doi:10.1080/00377317.2012.696984

Orcutt, B., & Mills, P. (1982). A model of doctoral education: Practice dimensions. In A. Rosen & J. Stretch (Eds.), *Doctoral education in social work: Issues, perspectives and evaluation* (pp. 3–10). St. Louis, MO: GADE.

Pearlman, C. (2013). Adjuncts in social work programs: Good practice or unethical? *Journal of Teaching in Social Work*, *33*, 209–219. doi:10.1080/08841233.2013.778939

Power, R., & Bogo, M. (2003). Educating field instructors and students to deal with challenges in their teaching relationships. *The Clinical Supervisor*, *21*, 39–58. doi:10.1300/J001v21n01_04

Prochaska, J., DiClemente, C., & Norcross, J. (1992). In search of how people change: Applications to addictive behaviors. *American Psychologist*, *47*, 1102–1114. doi:10.1037/0003-066X.47.9.1102

Raskin, M., & Blome, W. (1998). The impact of managed care on field instruction. *Journal of Social Work Education, 34*, 365–374.

Rubin, A. (2008). *Practitioner's guide to using research for evidence-based practice.* Hoboken, NJ: Wiley & Sons.

Saltzburg, S., Greene, G., & Drew, H. (2010). Using live supervision in field education: Preparing social work students for clinical practice. *Families in Society: The Journal of Contemporary Social Services, 91*, 293–299. doi:10.1606/1044-3894.4008

Schamess, G. (2012). Mutual influence in psychodynamic supervision. *Smith College Studies in Social Work, 82*, 142–160. doi:10.1080/00377317.2012.693012

Schilling, R., Morrish, J., & Liu, G. (2008). Demographic trends in social work over a quarter-century in an increasingly female profession. *Social Work, 53*, 103–114. doi:10.1093/sw/53.2.103

Shore, B. (1991). Is there a role for clinical doctoral education? No! *Journal of Social Work Education, 27*, 231–241.

Simpson, G., Williams, J., & Segall, A. (2007). Social work education and clinical learning. *Clinical Social Work Journal, 35*, 3–14. doi:10.1007/s10615-006-0046-4

Singer, J., & Greeno, C. (2013). When Bambi meets Godzilla. *Best Practices in Mental Health, 9*, 99–115.

Starr, R. (2007). Life, death, survival: Where goes our profession? [Message from the President.]. *Currents of the New York City Chapter, National Association of Social Workers, 52*(2), 2, 9, 10, 12.

Stegall, S., & Nangle, D. (2005). Successes and failures in the implementation of a manualized treatment for childhood depression in an outpatient setting. *Clinical Case Studies, 4*, 227–245. doi:10.1177/1534650103259718

Stoesz, S., Karger, H., & Carrilio, T. (2010). *A dream deferred: How social work education lost its way and what can be done about it.* New Brunswick, NJ: Aldine Transaction.

Tucker, D. (2003, January). *Empirical progress in social work scholarship: The role of theory.* Paper presented at the 2003 Conference for Society for Social Work and Research, Washington, DC.

United States Bureau of Labor Statistics. (2010–2011). *Occupational outlook handbook: Social workers 2010-2011.* Retrieved from http://www.bls.gov/ooh/community-and-social-service/social-workers.htm#tab-6

Urdang, E. (1991). The discipline of faculty advising. *Journal of Teaching in Social Work, 5*, 117–137. doi:10.1300/J067v05n01_10

Urdang, E. (1999). Becoming a field instructor: A key experience in professional development. *The Clinical Supervisor, 18*, 85–103. doi:10.1300/J001v18n01_06

Valentine, D., Edwards, S., Goghagan, D., Huff, M., Pereira, A., & Wilson, P. (1998). Preparing social work doctoral students for teaching: Report of a survey. *Journal of Social Work Education, 34*, 1–11.

Zastrow, C., & Bremner, J. (2004). Social work education responds to the shortage of persons with both a doctorate and a professional social work degree. *Journal of Social Work Education, 40*, 351–358.

# The "New" DSW Is Here: Supporting Degree Completion and Student Success

MERY DIAZ

*Department of Human Services, CUNY/New York City College of Technology, Brooklyn, New York, USA*

*Some have questioned whether there should be a practice doctorate in social work. Academics and other key stakeholders would appear to agree that the degree has a role within 21st-century social work practice and education. Practitioners increasingly seek out the degree, and current and emerging programs have developed to meet that demand. This article seeks to identify the characteristics of the new DSW students and their needs, and to target areas of support that DSW programs should provide for successful degree completion. These include financial assistance, academic rigor, and mentoring opportunities.*

## INTRODUCTION

The emergence of the new Doctorate in Social Work (DSW) degree has prompted much discussion regarding its relevance to the social work discipline, larger implications for doctoral education, and its place in the social work profession. Existing DSW programs are enrolling and graduating students, and new programs are under way. As such, students seeking DSW degrees (and those currently enrolled in these programs) require support for successful completion. Although very limited degree completion data from institutions currently granting DSW degrees are still not publicly available, existing evidence suggests that successful doctoral degree completion remains a challenge and student attrition continues at high rates (Hartocollis, Cnaan, Ledwith, 2014; Liechty, Liao, & Schull, 2009). For students in practice doctoral programs, who have traditionally funded their studies out of pocket, with little or no institutional or government funding (Anastas & Videka, 2012), identifying diverse support mechanisms becomes crucial. In addition, the need to fill vacancies on the faculties of the increasing number of BSW and MSW programs also has created urgency for doctoral-level graduates. Moreover, the characteristics of the new DSW students necessitate the delivery of institutional supports distinct from those required by their PhD peers. Considerations for funding, mentorship, dissertation support, and networking tailored to the structure of DSW programs and the career needs of their students must be addressed. As such, the aim of this article is to begin identifying the specific needs of DSW students and to identify areas of support that DSW programs can provide to students for successful degree completion. The article begins with a description the development of the "new" DSW, the status of existing programs, and projected career outcomes. Characteristics and needs of DSW students are then presented, followed by recommendations for additional areas of student support.

## THE EVOLUTION OF THE DSW

The current debate over the practice doctorate role, as an alternative to the traditional research doctorate, is complex and decades old. The first social work doctoral degrees (PhD) were awarded in the 1920s by Bryn Mawr College and the University of Chicago. The novel doctorate in social work (DSW), with coursework and program structure similar to the PhD, was developed and offered in the 1940s at the University of Pennsylvania, Catholic University, and Smith College. Soon after, most PhD-granting programs began to convert to the DSW degree. One hypothesis is that this shift was intended to elevate the status of the profession (Paulson, 2006). By the 1970s the number of DSW-granting programs overtook the number of PhD programs. Degrees from some programs, such as New York University, Smith College, and Simmons College, purported to be clinical degrees, contributing to the confusion over the DSW degree's function. That many in academic and research institutions held this degree furthered this blurring.

The demand for practice doctorates contributed to their continuity and to tensions in social work doctoral education. At one point it was reported that as many as 21 out of 48 doctoral programs in the United States and Canada were focusing on clinical or direct practice (Levin, 1991). However, during the 1990s a rapid conversion to PhDs began to take place—a shift suggesting strong efforts to cement a research identity in social work doctoral education and the diminished status of the DSW (Cnaan, Draine, & Dichter, 2008). With limited options, social workers began pursuing practice doctorates in related fields such as psychology, and from clinical programs developed by for-profit institutions and nonuniversity settings. Proponents of the PhD responded to the interest in the then-emerging practice doctorate programs and social workers' hope for professional and reimbursement parity with other mental health disciplines. Shore (1991) argued against the development of exclusively clinical doctoral programs and maintained that programs not based in universities made limited contributions to the improvement of practice while ultimately steering the profession away from a social welfare context. She also perceived the explicit focus on counseling as one that did not encompass the foundations of the social work profession and diverted attention from disadvantaged populations and from provision of services to a wider range of the population. With the field's consensus of this view forming during 1990s, practice doctorates all but disappeared.

More recently, however, practice doctorates have found renewed support across varied disciplines. Richardson (2006) argued for the role of practice doctorates in education as essential in bridging the gap between research and practice, and necessary for creating "stewards of the enterprise." Anastas and Videka (2012) valorized the development of "stewards of the enterprise" in social work, contending that social work should not be perceived solely as a discipline but also as a practice profession. Their position holds that doctoral education requires both "stewards of the discipline"—those who generate knowledge and are responsible for the field of educational study—and "stewards of the enterprise." The latter are concerned with attention to social work practice, service delivery, social policy, and social justice.

In her seminal book based on a national study of social work doctoral students, Anastas (2012) reported that many students perceived their doctoral programs to be more aligned with the culture of academia than with practice and that their own rich practice experience often was devalued. Existing PhD programs are perceived to have made only modest attempts, if any, to bridge the gap between research and practice, as they continue to prepare students primarily for research and academic careers. Many do not require MSW degrees for admission, speaking to a deprioritization of experiential knowledge in social work (Golde & Walker, 2006). All the while, the growth of BSW and MSW programs across the nation has created a challenge in recruiting doctoral-level faculty to teach practice courses, emphasizing the need for a new pedagogical focus in doctoral education (Anastas & Kuerbis, 2009; Zastrow & Brenner, 2004). However, the professional identity of social work is subject to compromise as we default to other professionals the practice of research in areas that have been commonly undertaken by social workers (Cournoyer & Adamek, 2001; O'Neill, 2000). Consequently, the historical rivalry between the DSW and PhD label is less salient than the need itself for more doctoral-level social work educators.

## "The Horse Is Already Out of the Barn"

Given the needs in the social work discipline, the emergence of a new DSW "practice doctorate" is increasingly garnering support and is now considered to have a place in the continuum of doctoral education (NASW, 2014). At the time of this writing, there are five universities currently pioneering the new DSW with somewhat different paradigms from its namesake: the University of Pennsylvania, the first of its kind; Rutgers University; the University of Tennessee-Knoxville; Aurora University; and a jointly sponsored program at St. Catherine University and the University of St. Thomas, that launched in August 2014. Two other programs are in the planning phase but have no publically available information: New York University, slated to launch in 2015 (J. Anastas, personal communication, May 26, 2014), and the University of Southern California (M. Nair, personal communication, May 27, 2014). As has been pointed out, it appears evident that people are willing to pay for an "accessible practice doctorate" (Anastas & Videka, 2012), and the apt DSW appears to fit the demand. As observers have noted, "the horse is already out of the barn" (NASW, 2014). For prospective students, these programs are made attractive by their accessibility for working professionals, with evening and weekend classes, distance learning features, and generally a shorter length of time for degree completion. For social work academic institutions, DSW programs may provide additional revenue streams. For the social work profession, these programs may ensure the availability of both "stewards of the discipline" and "stewards of the enterprise."

Overall, the new DSW programs' aim to prepare leading practitioners and scholars is an appropriate response to the changing needs of the profession, and therefore efforts should be taken to ensure that students successfully complete the degree. As of yet, not much is known about the types of students who enroll in these programs, and for now only one—the University of Pennsylvania—has graduates. It is unclear how these programs are delivering on their mission, how many students have completed the programs, or whether the programs have met their expectations for career outcomes. However, because the literature on doctoral education notes that many enrolled students fail to complete doctoral degrees, across all disciplines, supportive structures may be key to meeting the shared goal. Given the overall growth of the social work profession and the increasing need for doctoral graduates, it is imperative that DSW programs make special efforts to support their students' successful degree completion.

## DSW STUDENTS: WHAT WE KNOW AND DON'T KNOW

The increasing complexities of social work practice in today's sociopolitical and economic environment call for advanced social work training. Questions about the MSW's capacity to meet present practice challenges in the social work field, and in spite of mandatory continuing education requirements in all 50 states for licensure renewal, more formal university education may be needed. Historically, social workers specifically have sought advanced practice training in nonuniversity settings, more recently online programs, and in allied fields such as psychology (Anastas & Videka, 2012; Levin, 1991). The DSW, however, may emerge as a natural continuum for many seeking advanced training, and as such prompts our exploration of factors that may impact successful completion of this degree.

The limited literature on social work doctoral education focuses primarily on traditional PhD students and allows only for preliminary, but cautionary, inferences for DSW students. PhD programs, which have been almost exclusively research focused, have required a long-term commitment with an average of 7 years for completion. In this era of surmounting student debt, the length of time needed to complete the degree, of course, has significant financial implications. Not surprisingly, it has been noted that approximately 50% of doctoral students drop out before degree completion (Johnson, Green, & Kluever, 2000; Lovitts, 2001). This same study soberingly reported that social workers who earn doctoral degrees currently make up only 2% of all licensed social workers (Whitaker, Weismiller, & Clark, 2006). Additional issues in doctoral education highlight the increasing number of female students and the lack of student racial and cultural diversity. Even when social work produces more doctoral candidates from diverse backgrounds than any other similar field, there is still a serious lack of diversity among doctoral graduates, especially of African Americans (Anastas & Kuerbis, 2009; Zastrow & Brenner, 2004).

## Practice, Research, and Knowledge

Students attracted to practice doctorates understandably are said to be more concerned with practice development than with research (Lester, 2004). The appeal of professional doctorates may also be driven by students' abilities to focus on their own professional experiences and to use their own practice as a location for knowledge development (Fenge, 2009). Based on information from their websites, and an article published by Penn faculty, currently three of the operating DSW programs (Penn, Rutgers, and Tennessee) have missions that appeal to those wishing to advance clinical skills (Hartocollis et al., 2014). Aurora University's program and St. Catherine's and St. Thomas's DSW offer clinical doctorate with the aim of teaching in higher education, and Penn's program identifies preparation for university teaching as one of their goals.

An important note regarding direct practice is that although it is the most common form of practice among licensed social workers, the current complexities of the social work field may also call for advanced macrolevel training in doctoral education. At this time, none of the operating DSW programs explicitly identifies macrolevel practice education as part of its mission. The Leadership Forum and the Group for Advancement of Doctoral Education in Social Work (GADE) requested the development of a Task Force on Advanced Clinical Practice and during a 2011 meeting provided guidelines for DSW programs. One of the recommendations was for the development of a more encompassing "advanced practice doctorate" to account for a broad spectrum of need (Task Force on the DSW Degree, 2011).

Traditional PhDs largely have been seen as a research-based qualification undertaken primarily for obtaining a university post (Leonard, 2000). In contrast, students who undertake DSW studies are seeking advanced practice skills and may not seek faculty positions as a primary outcome of their studies. Nevertheless, this is a career option that might be pursued and encouraged in light of the shortage of doctoral faculty. Penn and Aurora cite preparation for university-level teaching. The St. Catherine and St. Thomas program states it is the first specifically designed for MSWs currently teaching at the bachelor's and master's level who are looking to advance their careers in university settings. These DSW programs have included the development of clinical scholarship and advanced practice skill building as part of their mission. The Penn and Aurora programs offer courses that focus on clinical research and teaching and others in research methodology and clinical measurement, and St. Catherine–St. Thomas also has designed a curriculum to address this aim. On their website, Rutgers notes, "Our curriculum bridges [this] gap by preparing practitioner-scholars to reconnect knowledge production with practice while they create new practitioner knowledge in the field" (http://dsw.socialwork.rutgers.edu/). Finally, Tennessee states, "The curriculum focuses on advanced clinical practice, clinical research and advanced practice leadership" (http://www.csw.utk.edu/dsw/) and offers modules on clinical research and applied statistics.

The dissertation is the culminating requirement of most doctoral programs and is deemed central to doctoral education because it certifies the candidates' ability for independent scholarship and becomes the beginning of their scholarly work (Anastas, 2012; Council of Graduate Schools, 2010). Lovitts (2001) posited that the dissertation should "reflect the training received, the technical skills, and the analytical and writing skills developed in a doctoral program" (p. 11). Although all DSW programs require the development and dissemination of knowledge for practice, only Penn and Aurora maintain the traditional dissertation requirement. The other three programs require capstone papers or "banded dissertations" (a nonempirical publishable paper, and a publishable paper based on the students' "clinical research"), design of a "clinical research project," or a case study that highlights theory-to-practice. Although the dissertation phase has been identified as a high-risk period of attrition for doctoral students across disciplines (Di Pierro, 2007), it begs the question if eliminating this long-standing scholarly requisite is the only logical alternative for the completion of DSW programs.

## Doctoral Student Demographics

Social work doctoral education, although more diverse than other disciplines, has been concerned about increasing the number of students from underrepresented ethnic and racial backgrounds. In a 2007 survey of doctoral students, Anastas (2012) reported that 67% of respondents identified as non-Hispanic Whites, 10.2% Black, 8.5% Hispanic, 7.1% Asian, 1.5% Native American, and 5.7% identified mixed race/ethnicity or not identified with the available categories. The Council on Social Work Education (CSWE) reports annual statistics on social work programs in the United States. The CSWE's survey of 73 doctoral social work programs in the United States that were members of GADE found that the proportion of newly enrolled students identifying with a historically underrepresented group was 39.8%. For full-time students currently taking coursework and having completed coursework, the percentages were 40.7% and 38.4%, respectively (CSWE, 2013). Many graduates report being in midlife and supporting dependents upon the onset of their doctoral studies (Anastas, 2012). It has been theorized that the later onset of doctoral studies may deter graduates from taking entry-level academic posts due to financial implications and family obligations (Anastas & Kuerbis, 2009; Karger & Stoesz, 2003; Lennon, 2005). Furthermore, a significantly high number of graduates have reported incurring debt loads anywhere between $30,000 and $43,430 for undergraduate and graduate, more than double the average debt since 1994. Students increasingly report that they self-fund their doctoral studies or required support from family, and taking on further loans (Anastas, 2012; Anastas & Kuerbis, 2009; Lowenberg, 1972). Student debt has become a national crisis, particularly debilitating for those who pursue professions such as social work and education, which are historically underpaid (Patton, 2012; Williams, 2014). With the exception of Penn's program, which reports having built an endowed scholarship fund, providing merit awards, and teaching assistantships, DSW programs do not appear ready or yet willing to provide adequate financial support for their students (NASW, 2014).

## DSW Program Structure

The existing and emerging DSW programs are structured to meet the needs of working professionals. It is expected that throughout their studies, students will be employed (and for most, *must be* employed) to finance their education. The programs require minimal time on campus, courses are structured as modules, and some use synchronous and asynchronous online technology for distance learning. Depending on the program, these features may allow some willing students to undertake interstate travel or even complete the program from across the nation. The programs also promote shorter time to degree completion than the traditional PhDs—anywhere from 3 to

5 years. This goal of rapid degree completion may be one reason why two of the programs forgo the formal dissertation requirement.

Finally, a note on entering students. Some of the programs organize their entering classes into cohorts. They are expected to attend classes and modules as a group, from entry to completion. These cohorts range from an average of 12–20 students. Course offerings include many electives, and the structure allows programs to hire additional "outside" faculty to teach. Anastas (2012) noted that this format has the advantage of recruiting eminent national faculty for short-term work but also brings the disadvantage that students are not expected to or likely to have opportunities for developing an apprenticeship relationship with core faculty in the manner of traditional PhD students. Doctoral education literature, however, has identified mentor and apprenticeship relationships between students and faculty as a key characteristic for promoting doctoral program completion and career development (Liechty et al., 2009; Smith, Maroney, Nelson, Abel, & Able, 2006; Jimenez, West, & Gokalp, 2011). Given the size of cohorts and the more limited time generally spent on campus, DSW students may be at a significant disadvantage in developing this critical element of their doctoral education, and the consequent acculturation and socialization into academia.

## Career Outcomes

A study by Anastas and Kuerbis (2009) reported that approximately 50–60% of doctoral graduates have academic jobs upon graduation. Almost one third of doctoral graduates obtained tenure-line faculty positions in CSWE-accredited programs (Anastas & Kuerbis, 2009). Another national study by the National Association of Social Workers (NASW) reported that only 32% of licensed social workers with a doctoral education held academic posts. In a 2014 publication Penn reported on the status of their DSW program. Since the first cohort was admitted in 2007, 71% of students have completed the program within three years, and 86% complete the program by year 5 (Hartocollis, et al., 2014). In her presentation, at SWPI, Dean Lina Hartocollis further elaborated that 20% of graduates were teaching full-time and 35% were teaching part-time. Evidence further speaking to the interest in higher education careers for those who pursue practice doctorates. The other programs present at the conference, Rutgers and Tennessee, were newer and did not yet have graduates. With the exclusion of the Aurora program, which projects degree completion in 5 years, all other programs project 3 years for degree completion.

## WHAT PROGRAMS NEED TO DO

The following are recommendations regarding what schools of social work could implement in order to support DSW students through their course of study. Based on the available doctoral social work education literature, areas for support have been identified as follows: clarifying goals for the degree and ensuring program quality, funding support for students, student mentorship and social networking, developing research skills, and considerations for ethical applications of distance learning.

## Clarifying Goals and Ensuring Quality

As DSW programs continue to evolve, it is critical that they begin paving the way toward a shared vision for their role within doctoral education. Evidenced by the convening of the DSW Task Force, organized by CSWE in 2011, and subsequent think thank organized by SWPI in the fall of 2013, the conversation about the role of the DSW among key stakeholders has begun. The dialogue and communication must continue, and should include practitioners who are interested in pursuing these advanced degrees, those who have obtained the DSW, and key leaders in the social work field who may welcome these advanced practitioners. Even as we experience low numbers of doctoral-level social workers, the aim is not to prepare social workers with advanced degrees for the sake of advanced degrees but because this goal prospectively meets the needs of the profession and has a valid place in specific leadership and academic roles. As the field itself becomes increasingly complex, globally expansive, and in need of sophisticated interventions and educators to address pervasive social problems, doctoral education should be organized to prepare students to meet these challenges. Clinical approaches are one aspect, but macroperspectives and interventions would also enrich the skill sets of advance practitioners. In addition, as BSW and MSW programs increasingly hire practice doctorate graduates, pedagogical training should be central in the DSW curriculum.

Taking lessons from other fields that have developed such doctorates, the DSW must be distinguishable from both the MSW and the traditional PhD. To this end, there may be a clear role for CSWE and GADE for providing accreditation and quality assurance, respectively. These steps can support gatekeeping and legitimacy for practice doctorate, particularly in health fields where doctoral-level practitioners are at the top of the hierarchy. Anastas and Videka (2012) additionally purported that having a practice doctorate located in CSWE accredited programs "is seen as a strategy for competing successfully with programs that lack grounding in social work practice skills and ethical standards" (p. 269).

Rutgers and Tennessee report acceptance rates of 40% and 50%, respectively (NASW, 2014). While Penn reports an average acceptance rate of 41% with 91% of those accepted, matriculating (Hartocollis et al., 2014). A primary mission of the programs is to prepare advanced practitioners, and although not all programs mandate a dissertation, they require publishable papers or scholarly capstone projects. To this extent, admission requirements need to be aligned with assessments that will likely predict writing competencies but should not override requirements aligned with practice wisdom. In this light, the GRE exam, which only the Tennessee program requires, can serve as a supplemental diagnostic qualification, always keeping in mind the exam's possible cultural bias. All the programs have a 2-year post-MSW experience requirement, but if clinical practice, advanced competencies, and leadership are primary goals for DSW graduates, this minimal practice requirement may need to be revisited.

## Research Skills and the Dissertation

Related to the mission of DSW programs, the dissertation requirement should be a standard requirement. The dissertation becomes an indisputable criterion of all doctoral education. Training in empirical work, the development of knowledge and the successful dissemination of knowledge are critical to the evolution of social work practice. To develop these competencies, research courses in DSW programs should not only address practice approaches (and the evidentiary literature behind them) but also quantitative and qualitative research methods, theory, and application. Research skills and knowledge development are distinctive requirements of doctoral education, and to expect less from DSW students places them at a significant disadvantage in relation to other mental health fields that have these standards of practice at the practice doctoral level (e.g., the PsyD). The Carnegie Foundation (Golde, Bueschel, Jones, & Walker, 2006, p. 22) stated that doctoral graduates must be able to "generate new knowledge and defend knowledge against claims and criticisms, conserve the most important ideas and findings that are the legacy of past and current work, and transform knowledge that has been generated and conserved by explaining and connecting it to ideas from other fields." In adapting this standard, DSW programs would be complying with the Task Force on the DSW Degree's (2011) recommendations that these must "clarify the distinction between the advanced master's level degree and the advanced practice doctorate," "clarify the purpose of the practice doctorate, including the core concepts and competencies," and "describe potential professional applications of the advanced practice doctorate in both direct practice and academic settings" (p. 4). Liechty and colleagues (2009) noted that 59% of attrition occurs in the first 2 years, suggesting that dissertation time largely accounts for the high attrition rate. Addressing this reality will involve manageable advisor-to-student ratios and providing students opportunities to be matched with faculty who share their same interests.

## Funding Support

As student debt continues to rise nationally and government aid is declining, a lack of financial resources has become a clear barrier to the completion of doctoral degrees. The emergence of the DSW creates a new revenue for social work programs but may contribute to unstable outcomes for students. Advancing the practice skills of social workers is critical, but if they are not supported in the process, the field will continue to experience a low rate of doctoral-level practitioners. Moreover, when universities primarily allocate funding to traditional PhD programs, while neglecting their DSW programs, they are sending an unequivocal message that practice oriented higher education is not a valued endeavor. In fact, unequal funding would go against the social justice values and ethics of the social work discipline to "ensure that all people have access to equal resources, services and opportunities they require to meet their basic human needs and to develop fully" (NASW, 2008).

DSW programs must work toward reducing economic barriers by ensuring that students are aware of grants and fellowships, actively recruiting funding for their studies, advocating that federal and state loan forgiveness programs include doctoral students, and seeking the development of research and teaching assistantships. Some BSW and MSW programs already are implementing efforts to increase the number of social work faculty holding doctoral and professional degrees by increasing the amount of money offered to candidates who have both a doctoral degree and a professional degree (Zastrow & Brenner, 2004). In addition, many programs are strongly advocating the payment of partial tuition, advocating loan forgiveness programs, and seeking external funding for their faculty to pursue advanced degrees. This provides a significant incentive, because many graduates (60%) intend to either pursue or return to academic posts (Anastas & Kuerbis, 2009). DSW programs can further advocate for the expansion of programs like the CSWE Minority Fellowship Fund aimed at supporting ethnic minority social work doctoral applicants.

## Mentorship and Social Networking Support

The educational literature strongly supports the role of mentorship and social network supports in promoting academic success and degree completion (Espinoza, 2006; Jimenez, West, & Gokalp, 2011; Lietchy et al., 2009; Smith et al., 2006). After completion of studies, doctoral students also must have opportunities to foster meaningful mentoring and professional relationships with faculty who have provided support and professional opportunities. Mentoring relationships provide students with introduction into the world of scholars and socialization into academia. Through these relationships students further their research interests and skills, as well as relationships with eminent leaders in the field. This is a particularly crucial area to support for women and students of color, who often are left to cope with less formal and less advantageous relationships when looking for support (Espinoza, 2006; Margolis & Romero, 1998).

## The Notion of Increasing Educational Access

Finally, as programs reconfigure their teaching structures with "innovative" pedagogical technologies that aim to expand access to those who would not otherwise have been able to pursue doctoral degrees, they should be cautioned about replacing traditional "bricks and mortar" and face-to-face educational interactions. Of the current DSW programs, the University of Tennessee, St. Catherine–St. Thomas University's are offered primarily online. More recently, Penn announced plans to restructure their program into a combined distance online/on-site format (L. Hartocollis, personal communication, February 24, 2015). Reamer (2013) wrote that online social work education, however, is associated with many ethical concerns. Limited research of the pedagogical validity of fully online programs, and the ability to teach practice skills through web-based formats, raises major questions for social work education. Reamer further highlighted social justice issues associated with online education, including inequitable Internet access, limited differentiated teaching tools for students with unique learning needs that may not be aligned with online formats, quality control issues of instruction and student integrity, and finally confidentiality. Another analysis of online learning notes that students from historically underrepresented groups show more limited achievement with online programs (Barnett, 2011; Meisenhelder, 2013). In addition, online education has been criticized for helping to create a two-tiered education system where only the elite will benefit from rich face-to-face environments.

For social work doctoral education, becoming scholars requires the exchange of ideas and dynamic interactions between student and teacher, and student and student, especially because of the interpersonal nature of social work. Related fields have taken a similarly cautionary stance on online education. In 2010, following a period of public comment, the American Psychological Association's (APA's) Commission on Accreditation adopted an implementing regulation that prohibits doctoral programs that are primarily or completely online from being APA accredited (APA, 2008).

## CONCLUSION AND RECOMMENDATIONS

There is still very limited data about current DSW students. Future research should seek to gain a further understanding about who they are, their reasons for pursuing a doctoral degree, and how they differ (if they do) from PhD students. It is important to assess unique challenges faced in completing these programs and what incentives are present for completion. As the few existing programs continue to generate graduates, and new programs emerge, employment outcomes, for example, must be explored. This is relevant not only with respect to the career options for graduates but to understand how the DSW degree is being perceived in both practice and academic settings.

Within social work the question of whether there should be a practice doctorate appears to no longer be relevant. The answer appears to be "yes," as educators and other key stakeholders continue to dialogue about the place the degree should occupy within 21st-century social work practice and education, as candidates increasingly seek out the degree, and as emerging programs develop to meet that demand.

As noted, the development of the new DSW has several goals. The degree intends to prepare doctoral-level graduates who will bridge the gap between research and practice and fill the increasing number of university faculty positions. Furthermore, the DSW aims to address the need for advanced social work practice and supervisory skills in an ever more complicated social context for agency-based practice. Yet, in an era of rising student debt, considerations must be given to the kinds of supports available for DSW students. Programs should urgently consider the challenges created by rising tuition and the period to degree completion. Other critical considerations include academic rigor, dissertation support, and the development of strong mentorship and network relationships, widely considered essential resources in ensuring student success in doctoral education.

# REFERENCES

American Psychological Association. (2008). *Implementing regulations frequently used in program review*. Retrieved from http://www.apa.org/ed/accreditation/about/policies/implementing-regulations.aspx

Anastas, J. (2012). *Doctoral education in social work*. New York, NY: Oxford University Press.

Anastas, J. W., & Kuerbis, A. N. (2009). Doctoral education in social work: What we know and what we need to know. *Social Work, 54*, 71–81. doi:10.1093/sw/54.1.71

Anastas, J., & Videka, L. (2012). Does social work need a "practice doctorate"? *Clinical Social Work Journal, 40*, 268–276. doi:10.1007/s10615-012-0392-3

Barnett, E. (2011). Validation experiences and persistence among community college students. *The Review of Higher Education, 34*(2), 193–230.

Cnaan, R. A., Draine, J., & Dichter, M. E. (2008). Introduction: An overview of the journey. In R. A. Cnaan, J. Draine, & M. E. Dichter (Eds.), *A century of social work and social welfare at Penn* (pp. 1–9). Philadelphia, PA: Penn Press.

Council of Graduate Schools. (2010). *Ph.D. completion and attrition: Policy, numbers, leadership, and next steps*. Washington, DC: Author.

Council on Social Work Education. (2008). *Education policy and accreditation standards*. Alexandria, VA: Author.

Council on Social Work Education. (2013). *Annual statistics on social work education in the United States*. Retrieved from http://www.cswe.org/File.aspx?id=74478

Cournoyer, B. R., & Adamek, M. E. (2001). The 2001 educational policy and accreditation standards: The value of research revisited. *Advances in Social Work, 2*, 119–126.

Di Pierro, M. (2007). Excellence in doctoral education: Defining best practices. *College Student Journal, 47*, 368–375.

Espinoza, R. M. (2006). *Timing of pivotal moments and graduate school social support networks among Whites, Latinas, and African Americans.* Paper presented at the annual meeting of the American Sociological Association, Montreal, Quebec. Retrieved from http://citation.allacademic.com/meta/p104530_index.html

Fenge, L. (2009). Professional doctorates-a better route for researching professionals? *Social Work Education, 28*, 165–176. doi:10.1080/02615470701865733

Golde, C. M., Bueschel, A. C., Jones, L., & Walker, G. E. (2006). *Apprenticeship and intellectual community: Lessons from the Carnegie Initiative on the Doctorate.* Retrieved from http://www.ilr.cornell.edu/sites/ilr.cornell.edu/files/Apprenticeship%20and%20Intellectual%20Community%20Lessons%20from%20the%20Carnegie%20Initiative%20on%20the%20Doctorate.pdf

Golde, C. M., & Walker, G. E. (Eds.). (2006). *Envisioning the future of doctoral education: Preparing stewards of the discipline.* San Francisco, CA: Jossey-Bass.

Hartocollis, L., Cnaan, R. A., & Ledwith, K. (2014). The social work practice doctorate. *Research on Social Work Practice, 24*(5), 636–642.

Jimenez, Y., West, I., & Gokalp, G. (2011). Effective strategies for supporting doctoral students. *The International Journal of Diversity in Organizations, Communities and Nations, 11*, 11–20.

Johnson, E. M., Green, K. E., & Kluever, R. C. (2000). Psychometric characteristics of the revised procrastination inventory. *Research in Higher Education, 41*, 269–279. doi:10.1023/A:1007051423054

Karger, H. S., & Stoesz, D. (2003). The growth of social work education programs, 1985–1999; its impact on economic and education factors related to the profession of social work. *Journal of Social Work Education, 39*, 279–295.

Lennon, T. M. (2005). *Statistics on social work education in the United States: 2003.* Alexandria, VA: Council on Social Work Education.

Leonard, D. (2000). Transforming doctoral studies: Competencies and artistry. *Higher Education in Europe, 25*, 181–192. doi:10.1080/713669254

Lester, S. (2004). Conceptualizing the practitioner doctorate. *Studies in Higher Education, 29*, 757–770. doi:10.1080/0307507042000287249

Levin, A. (1991). Is there a role for clinical doctoral education? Yes! *Journal of Social Work Education, 27*, 235–238.

Liechty, J. M., Liao, M., & Schull, C. P. (2009). Facilitating dissertation completion and success among doctoral students in social work. *Journal of Social Work Education, 45*, 481–497. doi:10.5175/JSWE.2009.200800091

Lovitts, B. E. (2001). *Leaving the ivory tower: The causes and consequences of departure from doctoral study.* Lanham, VA: Rowman & Littlefield.

Lowenberg, F. M. (1972). *Doctoral students in social work.* New York: Council on Social Work Education.

Margolis, E., & Romero, M. (1998). "The department is very male, very white, very old, and very conservative": The functioning of the hidden curriculum in graduate sociology departments. *Harvard Educational Review, 68*, 1–32.

Meisenhelder, S. (2013). MOOC mania. *Thought and Action, 29*, 7–26.

National Association of Social Workers. (2008). *NASW Code of ethics.* Washington, DC: Author.

National Association of Social Workers. (2014). *Social Work Policy Institute: Advanced practice doctorates: What do they mean for social work practice, research, and education.* Retrieved from http://www.socialworkpolicy.org/wp-content/uploads/2014/01/SWPI_DSW_FINAL_Report.pdf

O'Neill, J. V. (2000). Larger doctoral enrollments sought: Few social workers follow path to PhD [Electronic version]. *NASW News.* November. Retrieved from http://www.socialworkers.org/pubs/news/2000/11/phd.htm

Patton, S. (2012). *The Ph.D. now comes with food stamps.* Retrieved from http://chronicle.com/article/from-Graduate-School-to/131795

Paulson, D. (2006, June). *Catholic university retroactively confers PhD on DSW graduates.* GWSCSW News and Views. P.5. Retrieved from http://www.gwscsw.org/PDFs/2006_06NV.pdf

Reamer, F. G. (2013). Distance and online social work education: Novel ethical challenges. *Journal of Teaching in Social Work, 33,* 369–384. doi:10.1080/08841233.2013.828669

*Report of the Task Force on the DSW Degree Convened by the Social Work Leadership Forum.* (2011). Retrieved from http://www.cswe.org/File.aspx?id=59954

Richardson, V. (2006). Stewards of a field, stewards of an enterprise: The doctorate in education. In C. M. Golde & G. E. Walker (Eds.), *Envisioning the future of doctoral education: Preparing stewards of the discipline* (pp. 251–267). San Francisco, CA: Jossey-Bass.

Shore, B. K. (1991). Is there a role for clinical doctoral education? No! *Journal of Social Work Education, 27*(3), 239–241.

Smith, R. L., Maroney, K., Nelson, K. W., Abel, A. L., & Able, H. S. (2006). Doctoral programs: Changing high rates of attrition. *The Journal of Humanistic Counseling, Education and Development, 45,* 17–31. doi:10.1002/j.2161-1939.2006.tb00002.x

Social Work Policy Institute. (2013). *Advanced practice doctorates: What do they mean for social work practice, research, and education.* Retrieved from http://www.socialworkpolicy.org/wp-content/uploads/2014/01/SWPI_DSW_FINAL_Report.pdf

Task Force on the DSW Degree. (2011). *The doctorate in social work (DSW) degree: Emergence of a new practice doctorate report of the task force on the DSW degree convened by the social work leadership forum.* Retrieved from http://www.naddssw.org/pages/wp-content/uploads/2009/09/DSW-Degree-Task-Force-Report-April-16-2011.pdf

Whitaker, T., Weismiller, T., & Clark, E. (2006). *Assuring the sufficiency of a frontline workforce: A national study of licensed social workers* (Executive summary). Washington, DC: National Association of Social Workers.

Williams, A. (2014). *The cost of a Ph.D.: Students report hefty debt across many fields.* Retrieved from http://chronicle.com/article/The-Cost-of-a-PhD-Students/144049

Zastrow, C., & Brenner, J. (2004). Social work education responds to the shortage of persons with both a doctoral and a professional social work degree. *Journal of Social Work Education, 40,* 351–358.

# An Evaluation of the University of Pennsylvania's Practice Doctorate (DSW) Program

LINA HARTOCOLLIS, PHYLLIS SOLOMON, ANDREA DOYLE,
and MATTHEW DITTY

*School of Social Policy & Practice, University of Pennsylvania, Philadelphia,
Pennsylvania, USA*

*This article reports on an evaluation of the University of Pennsylvania's doctorate in social work (DSW), the first of the newly emerging practice doctorates. The study sample was current students and program alumni. Data were from program records and from an online survey of DSW alumni with an 81.6% response rate. Overall, the program is achieving its explicit and implicit goals. Current students and alumni are being hired part-time and full-time to teach in BSW and MSW programs. Moreover, graduates have found that the degree enhanced their recognition and respect by colleagues and professionals from other disciplines and resulted in greater confidence from clients.*

The emerging practice doctorate in social work (DSW) is in a phase of active development and refinement. Since the University of Pennsylvania introduced the DSW prototype in 2007, other social work programs also have begun offering the practice doctorate alongside the research-based PhD. The reemergence of the DSW, specifically as a practice doctorate, has started a discipline-wide conversation about the identity, purpose, and value of this new credential and its potential impact on the social work education and practice landscape (Anastas & Videka, 2012; Nurius & Kemp, 2014; Social Work Policy Institute, 2013). This study provides a program description along with a summative evaluation of the University of Pennsylvania's DSW program, based on data collected from program records and an online survey conducted with alumni of the program.

Social work is a relative latecomer to the practice doctorate enterprise, following other professions, namely, psychology (Peterson, 1997), nursing (Buchholz et al., 2013; Starck, Duffy, & Vogler, 1993), education (Maxwell, 2003), occupational therapy (Pierce & Peyton, 1999), physical therapy (Threlkeld, Jensen, & Royeen, 1999), and pharmacy (Talbert, 1997), several of which have moved to requiring the doctorate as the terminal degree for professional practice (Bollag, 2007; Shulman, Golde, Bueschel, & Garabedian, 2006). However, even in social work the practice doctorate is not a new idea, having been proposed and debated since the 1970s (Donahoe, 2000; Shore & Levin, 1991). In 1978, the late William Reid called for a practice doctorate that would arm clinical social workers with the credentials to obtain third-party payments, better agency positions, and higher salaries (Reid, 1978). Levin specifically saw the clinical doctorate as a means to enhance clinical training, improve the status of the profession, and promote greater professional acceptance and heightened career satisfaction (Shore & Levin, 1991).

Shortly after Reid made his public appeal for a practice doctorate, the Russell Sage Foundation began infusing money into social work doctoral programs to kick-start a more scientific base to the discipline, leading away from a preoccupation with practitioner concerns (such as casework processes) in favor of measurable outcomes (Doyle, 2011). More recently, there has been a general push in the field for elevating the social work research enterprise to a science (Brekke, 2012; Fong, 2012) and for producing generalizable knowledge (Thyer, 1997), traditionally the concern and purview of the PhD.

Now that several DSW programs have been launched in addition to the University of Pennsylvania—at the time of this writing at Rutgers University, University of Tennessee, and Aurora University—and a number of others are in the pipeline, the conversation has turned from whether the profession should have a practice doctorate to what the practice doctorate means for the profession and how to ensure quality and accountability (Anastas & Videka, 2012). In 2011, the Council on Social Work Education (CSWE) convened a task force that produced a set of "quality guidelines" (Task Force on the DSW Degree, 2011). In the fall of 2013, a 2-day "invitational think tank" on the advanced practice doctorate was convened in Washington, DC, by the National Association of Social Workers, the CSWE, the National Association of Deans and Directors of Schools of Social Work, the Association of Baccalaureate Social Work Program Directors, the Group for the Advancement of Doctoral Education in Social Work, the Society for Social Work and Research, the St. Louis Group for Excellence in Social Work Research and Education, and the Association of Social Work Boards, which brought together stakeholders to consider how practice doctorates fit with the overall practice and research mission of the social work profession. The proceedings were summarized in a report titled "Advanced Practice Doctorates: What Do They Mean for Social Work Practice, Research and Education." Among the report's recommendations was to develop scholarship about the existing DSW programs, including outcomes such as impact on the career mobility of graduates (Social Work Policy Institute, 2013).

## HISTORY AND RATIONALE OF THE PENN DSW PROGRAM

For many years the PhD in social work and the DSW were considered essentially interchangeable; as Thyer (2002) noted, both were "usually research oriented academic degrees, not clinically oriented ones" (p. 6). By the late 1990s, the DSW was on the decline, with only a few programs still offering the degree (Thyer, 2002). Following this trend, the University of Pennsylvania discontinued its original DSW degree in the 1990s and moved to offering only the PhD (Cnaan, Draine, & Dichter, 2008).

By 2007 there were no longer any DSW programs in the country, which presented an opportunity to reinvent the degree as a practice doctorate. The decision to reintroduce the University of Pennsylvania's DSW as a professional practice doctorate—intended to prepare students for advanced clinical practice and teaching, and clearly differentiated from the PhD—came in response to four areas of perceived need: (a) to generate new clinical social work knowledge; (b) to advance the evidence-based expertise of social work practitioners; (c) to prepare doctoral-level practitioner-scholars who disseminate social work practice knowledge through teaching, presentation, scholarship, and practice; and (d) to enhance the professional status of social work practitioners.

Several troubling trends in doctoral education were taken into account while planning the University of Pennsylvania's DSW. Of particular concern was the shortage of doctoral-trained faculty to teach in BSW and MSW programs, especially those who hold the MSW and have sufficient postmaster's practice experience (Zastrow & Bremner, 2004) to qualify them to teach practice according to CSWE accreditation requirements (CSWE Commission on Accreditation, 2012; Johnson & Munch, 2010). The significant proportion of PhD graduates who choose employment outside the academy (Anastas, 2012; Khinduka, 2002) suggested that some were choosing the PhD, even though the stated purpose of the degree did not fit with their career goals, simply because it was the only option available for social work doctoral study. In a similar vein, the lack of a social work practice doctorate was leading many MSWs to pursue doctoral degrees in other related professions. The risk that the social work profession would be left behind, as other professions adopted practice doctorates, was also a concern, as social workers in multidisciplinary settings frequently were the only ones at the table who were not qualified and titled as doctors. Furthermore, there was growing awareness of the practice–research divide and the need for more applied practice research and scholarship that would be readily available, accessible, and relevant to front line practitioners (Austin, 1997; Brekke, Ell, & Palinka, 2007; Fong & Pomeroy, 2011).

The problem of high noncompletion rates in PhD programs, with many doctoral students not finishing the dissertation and remaining "all but dissertation" (Anastas, 2012; Denecke & Frasier, 2005; Shulman, 2010), was taken into account when designing Penn's DSW program. In addition, the practical realities that make full-time doctoral study inaccessible for working professionals (who cannot afford to leave their jobs) were considered. As noted next in the program description, the course schedule and dissertation work were carefully structured to be convenient for working professionals, and doable within the time frame set out for degree completion.

## PROGRAM GOALS

The DSW goals, which drove the program's initial design and serve as touchstones for ongoing program evaluation and continuous improvement, are as follows. To produce graduates who (a) are able to critically analyze and apply a range of social, behavioral, and practice theories and models; (b) are capable of designing and implementing empirically grounded clinical social work interventions; (c) are critical consumers of clinical research and able to conduct sound, evidence-based inquiry on issues of significance to social work practice; (d) are content experts with deep knowledge in at least one chosen area related to social work practice and who disseminate this knowledge through teaching, presentation, practice, and scholarly activities; and (e) are competent educators who are able to teach and engage in course and curriculum development. In addition to these explicit goals, implicit goals included high completion rates and reasonably short time frame to degree, and among graduates, increased professional status, career mobility, and opportunities for advancement.

## PROGRAM DESCRIPTION

The University of Pennsylvania's DSW program is tailored to balance the rigor of a doctoral degree with the logistical considerations of busy working professionals in the field; it is structured as an intensive 3-year course of study consisting of classroom learning, directed individual study, faculty mentoring, and opportunities for gaining classroom teaching experience. All of the classes are taught on campus, and students are required to be physically present; there are no online courses offered. The cohort effect is a central pedagogical strategy and is supported by keeping students together throughout the program, building in time for socializing and interaction among students and faculty, such as breaks between classes and group meals. This would be difficult to do with a distance learning format.

The core curriculum in the 1st year consists of two semester-length classes on applied clinical theory and two semester-length research methods classes. Students take an applied social statistics course that exposes them to statistical methods that are commonly used in social work research, which equips them to choose appropriate methods of statistical analysis if they plan to undertake a quantitative or mixed method dissertation. During the 1st year, courses meet one late afternoon/evening each week.

Upon completion of the first two semesters, students are required to pass a preliminary examination to determine eligibility to continue in the program. Until 2013, the format of the preliminary exam was an open-book take-home test that obliged students to respond to essay questions related to the content from the 1st-year core classes. In 2014, the DSW governance committee changed the format of the exam to a critical review of the literature related to the student's dissertation topic, which must be completed and approved by the dissertation chair by the fall semester of Year 2, after which the student may advance to the dissertation proposal stage.

Beginning in the summer following the 1st year of study, classes are taught in monthly weekend "modules" that begin Fridays and continue through Saturday. The module structure is convenient for the students, most of whom are working full-time, and allows for bringing in preeminent faculty and clinician experts from all over the country. The course modules are organized around topical areas related to social work practice and teaching, such as trauma-informed care, substance abuse practice, interventions with youth, outcomes measurement, statistics, cultural competence, group work, relational theory, dialectical behavior therapy, and teaching. In addition to the courses on teaching in the curriculum, students may serve as teaching assistants in the MSW program after completing their 1st year of study, and those with teaching experience are eligible to serve as part-time instructors and teach a maximum of one class each semester in the MSW program.

The coursework and dissertation are conducted simultaneously and completed concurrently, in contrast to the traditional PhD model of coursework, followed by the dissertation. This time-limited, highly structured program design was intended to address the completion rate problem that is endemic in PhD programs in social work and sister disciplines (Anastas, 2012; Denecke & Frasier, 2005; Shulman, 2010). In the PhD, the open-ended dissertation serves as something of a proving ground and launching pad to demonstrate a candidate's suitability for a career in the academy where autonomous scholarly productivity is the sine qua non. Because the goal of the DSW is to produce clinician-scholars who, if they choose to teach, are likely to either combine practice and part-time teaching or serve as faculty in teaching-oriented settings, the dissertation process is tightly structured and time limited, with the twin goal of producing high-quality scholarly work and finishing on time.

Students are provided with ample writing and mentoring support to promote timely degree completion. In addition to the typical dissertation committee, each student is assigned a dissertation mentor who spends the 1st year (before the dissertation committee is assembled) helping the student to decide on a topic and narrow in on a relevant and appropriately scaled research question. Another key source of support and structure built into the program is the cohort model, whereby each group of 15 entering students stays together, taking all classes as a cohort throughout the 3 years of the program. As Shulman (2010) noted in his argument that PhD programs would do well to borrow from the professional doctorates as they tackle the low completion rate,

> the cohort effect—the influence of other students in the same class who form a learning community of support and critique—is generally much more powerful in the professions because of the way in which a group of candidates stays together, sharing each point in its education. (p. B11)

Shulman noted that "the open-endedness of doctoral education has become one of its deepest flaws" (p. B10).

Students in Penn's DSW program may produce either a traditional book-style dissertation or an article-style dissertation that employs one of the following methods or formats: empirical study (quantitative, qualitative, or mixed methods), curriculum development, historical analysis, conceptual/theoretical analysis, adaptation or development of an intervention, or a program evaluation. The dissertation serves two purposes that follow directly from the DSW program's mission and goals: (a) to enable students to become content experts, gaining deep knowledge in an area of practice, and (b) to be able to make a contribution to the social work practice knowledge base. This latter purpose is achieved by publishing the dissertations on Scholarly Commons, an open source electronic repository for scholarship hosted by the University of Pennsylvania.

## STUDENT DESCRIPTION

Admission to the University of Pennsylvania's DSW program is selective. The average number of applicants per year is 32, for a class of 15 students. The average admission yield is 91%, calculated as the percentage of admitted

**TABLE 1** University of Pennsylvania Doctorate in Social Work Student and Alumni Characteristics

|  | Students and graduates[a] | | Alumni survey respondents[b] | |
|---|---|---|---|---|
|  | n | % | n | % |
| Race/Ethnicity | | | | |
| White | 64 | 60.0 | 25 | 62.5 |
| African American/Black | 25 | 23.8 | 9 | 22.5 |
| Asian | 7 | 06.7 | 4 | 10.0 |
| Hispanic/Latino | 2 | 01.9 | 2 | 05.0 |
| Multiple | 8 | 07.6 | 0 | 0.0 |
| Gender | | | | |
| Female | 88 | 83.0 | 34 | 85.0 |
| Male | 18 | 17.0 | 6 | 15.0 |
| Age | $M = 37$ $(SD = 9)$ | | $M = 42$ $(SD = 9.2)$ | |
| Range | 25–61 | | 30–61 | |

[a]$N = 106.$ [b]$N = 40.$

applicants who accept the offer of admission. Qualified applicants must hold a master of social work degree from an accredited program and have at least 2 years' postmaster's experience. However, the average length of postmaster's practice experience of students who enter the program is considerably greater, with a mean of 7.5 years and a range of 2 to 18 years.

To date, the program has admitted 106 students who are close to two thirds Caucasian, almost one fourth African American, and predominately female. The mean age is 37 ($SD = 9$) with a range from 25 to 61 (see Table 1). The student draw is primarily regional, with most commuting in from Pennsylvania, New Jersey, New York, District of Columbia, Delaware, Maryland, and Virginia. However, some students have commuted from as far away as Connecticut and Maine, and students have relocated from Boston, South Carolina, Ohio, California, and Michigan to attend the program.

The retention rate of the program is 91%. Of the 106 students who began the program, three students withdrew voluntarily, all of them during the 1st year of the program; three students requested and were granted leaves of absence for personal or health reasons; and four students were dismissed during or directly following the 1st year of the program for failure to maintain satisfactory academic progress.

## SUMMATIVE EVALUATION

### Methods

*Design.* The outcome assessment of the program was based on data collected from program records, on the university's electronic warehouse of student data, and from an online survey. The online survey was distributed in December, 2013 and resent January 2014 via e-mail to all alumni of the program. (The survey was conducted as part of an outcome evaluation of the DSW program and therefore was not research; hence, Institutional Review Board approval was not sought.) Forty-nine graduates were surveyed, with a response rate of 81.6% ($N = 40$). The survey contained both closed-ended and open-ended questions. The closed-ended questions entailed basic demographic information. The open-ended questions comprised scholarly activities in which alumni were engaged, such as positions held, at which institution, what classes taught, and whether they had published or presented at professional meetings during or after graduation from the DSW program. In addition, they were asked for a personal assessment of the impact of the DSW program on their career, such as age. "How did the DSW program help you with your job? For example, were you promoted internally or given additional responsibilities, did you receive additional recognition, were you able to apply knowledge or research skills from DSW study, etc. Please be specific."

*Analysis.* The close-ended responses were tallied and converted to percentages for categorical data, and descriptive statistics were employed when appropriate, consisting mostly of means. For open-ended responses, the answers were independently read by two of the authors and each extracted themes. The two then compared themes to determine consensus. There was 100% agreement, with some additional elaboration of a given theme. The Word Cloud procedure was used to validate the themes extracted by the two (see Figure 1). This procedure employs a word count tally from the text and displays the size of terms based on their frequency.

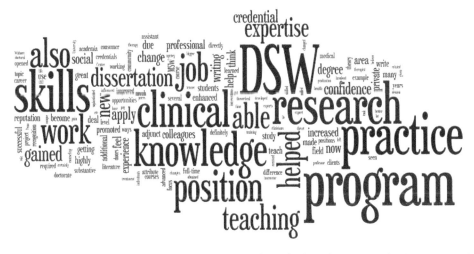

**FIGURE 1** Assessment of the doctorate in social work (DSW) program by University of Pennsylvania alumni.

## Description of Alumni Survey Respondents

The average age of respondents was 42, with a range from 30 to 61. The sample was predominately female and Caucasian, with almost one fourth identifying themselves as Black/African American (see Table 1). The sample well represented the current students and graduates demographically. The alumni mean age of respondents was 5 years older than the general student population. Almost all were employed when they began the program. A number described themselves as private practitioners, psychotherapists, and clinical social workers/therapists, whereas a smaller number indicated they held administrative positions, such as assistant project director, director of transition services, or technical director. Ninety-five percent of respondents stated that they continued working throughout the program.

## Findings: Program Impact and Outcomes

Nine major themes evolved from the responses to the open-ended questions (see Table 2). The most predominant theme that emerged from alumni respondents, which was consistent with program goals, was that as result of the program they had improved their practice knowledge and skills and had enhanced their confidence in their practice competencies. This theme is evident in Figure 1, where the relative size of the word represents the frequency of its use by respondents.

As one responded stated,

> It helped me to be a stronger social work practitioner/clinician in that I was surrounded by other strong practitioners/clinicians, and I was able to integrate and apply a great deal of information and knowledge from the course materials/class discussions. The process was greatly enhanced by having faculty who brought a great deal of experience and were highly skilled in their own right.

**TABLE 2** Themes of Program Impact From University of Pennsylvania Doctorate in Social Work (DSW) Alumni Respondents

| | |
|---|---|
| 1 | Improved practice, knowledge, skills, and confidence—am stronger social work practitioner/clinician |
| 2 | Enhanced research skills—greater understanding and use of research—engaged in doing research and evaluation |
| 3 | Helped refine writing and thinking skills—adding scholarly writing to my professional life |
| 4 | Gained in-depth expertise—"intellectually nourishing & professionally stimulating" |
| 5 | Enabled obtaining teaching positions, or teaching courses—mixing teaching with practice |
| 6 | Increased responsibilities and more responsible job |
| 7 | Greater recognition and respect from peers and colleagues from other disciplines; increased confidence and credibility with clients/patients |
| 8 | No change; DSW not seen as asset; no opportunity to be promoted in organization |

Also in line with program goals, a number of respondents mentioned that the program enhanced their research skills, as well as their understanding and use of research. Some commented on the fact that they were now actually engaged in conducting research and evaluation. A few further stated that the expertise gained in producing their dissertation increased their credibility with others and improved their practice. A statement by one respondent captures this theme:

> Learning about research methods and then completing my own research project for my dissertation has made a profound difference in many ways in my career. I feel like I understand science and use science more in my practice. I have become a much more sophisticated consumer of research.

Consistent with the program goal of disseminating knowledge through engagement in scholarly activities, some respondents stated that the program helped refine their writing and thinking skills and that scholarship became a part of their professional life. One even noted being surprised by liking scholarly writing so much.

Students and graduates have produced published scholarship and presented at professional conferences, in keeping with the program goal of facilitating knowledge creation and dissemination. Students have had professional articles accepted for publication in journals such as *Clinical Social Work Journal, Psychoanalytic Social Work, Social Work in Health Care*, and *Journal of Prevention and Intervention in the Community*. Several students have co-authored book chapters, one student's dissertation was published as a book, one program graduate co-authored an instructor's manual for clinical social work practice in behavioral health, and another co-edited a professional textbook. In response to the survey, alumni also reported presenting at numerous professional conferences, including the Society for Social Work and Research and the Council on Social Work Education APM.

As further evidence of positive outcomes with respect to the goal of facilitating knowledge creation and dissemination, at the time of this writing the 47 DSW dissertations had been downloaded more than 60,000 times from Scholarly Commons, the university's publically accessible repository for scholarly work.

Related to the theme of knowledge acquisition and development was the expertise that respondents felt they had gained, often from the dissertation work, which they found to be "intellectually nourishing and professionally stimulating" and from which they garnered recognition, as there often was a dearth of empirical evidence in their domain of research. Some noted that they felt better equipped to work with specific client populations. One specifically stated feeling like a "better supervisor" as a result of the program.

Some respondents noted that having the doctorate increased their credibility and prestige. One elaborated that because the degree came from an Ivy League institution, it had resulted in increased recognition and respect from peers and colleagues, such as psychiatrists. The respondent also described how the status conferred by the DSW credential led clients/patients to have greater confidence in the respondent's clinical ability. As one stated,

> My research was related to my area of specialty. I believe it added to my cache as a specialist in my area. I presented at numerous conferences about the research. It was the first study of its kind and that impacted my reputation in the field.

Others indicated that as a result of the program, they were able to gain additional job responsibilities, promotions, or new jobs, some of which they would not have been eligible for without the doctoral degree. Specifically, a number of the respondents stated that they were able to obtain full-time teaching positions, or teach courses on a part-time basis, and that this was made possible by their doctoral degree. A few specified that they were now able to blend teaching with their practice. One respondent specifically noted, "I would not have had the confidence to teach in an MSW program before getting my DSW and certainly would not have known how to design my own course." It is important to note that graduates are teaching a variety of courses at both the BSW and MSW level, from research methods, human behavior and the social environment, diversity, and mental health diagnosis to practice courses that focus on particular interventions or populations. An additional respondent described an opportunity to teach medical residents. However, there were a few who noted no change in position or responsibilities after earning the DSW. One stated that her agency did not see the program as an "asset," whereas another noted that there was not an opportunity for upward mobility but was carrying a very responsible position already.

A goal of the University of Pennsylvania's DSW program is to address the low doctorate degree completion rate by providing a tightly structured, time-limited curriculum. With respect to completion rates and time to degree, 71% of the program's graduates finished the degree requirements by Year 3 and 86% by Year 5. This compares favorably to the 60% completion rate for PhDs in all disciplines (including the social sciences) by Year 10 and the completion rate for social work PhDs of 66.7% by Year 7 (Sowell, 2008).

## CONCLUSION, DISCUSSION, AND RECOMMENDATIONS

Based on program data and survey responses, the University of Pennsylvania's DSW program clearly is achieving its stated goals. Although the jury is still out on the long-term direction and impact of the nascent social work practice doctorate, the preliminary results reported here suggest that the DSW holds promise as a value-added option alongside the PhD. Penn DSW graduates are applying what they learned in the program to enhance and critically evaluate their own practice, and social work practice generally. They have furthermore become better consumers and utilizers of existing practice evidence. Graduates are helping to fill a critical need for doctoral-level practice teachers in BSW and MSW programs with current students and alumni being hired as full-time practice professors and part-time faculty in BSW, MSW, and other human service programs. Consistent with Levin's argument in 1991 (Shore & Levin, 1991), graduates are reporting that they have gained recognition and credibility by virtue of having the DSW credential, which for some has translated into opportunities for career advancement and new career opportunities. At least two program graduates have successfully competed for jobs with doctoral-level candidates from other disciplines, namely, psychology and nursing.

An unexpected finding was how valuable the students perceived the dissertation. Alumni reported liking and appreciating the dissertation work more than they had expected. Some noted that it enhanced their ability to work with specific client populations, which echoes Levin's words: "Dissertation experience significantly affects their clinical practice in a positive way" (Shore & Levin, 1991, p. 236). The disciplined dissertation process and faculty mentoring gave students the confidence to publish and write, positioned them as content experts, and led to increased recognition and career mobility. Through the dissertation, professional publications, and presentations, students and graduates are producing scholarship in areas that had not previously been well addressed in the clinical literature.

Of the four DSW programs currently in existence, the University of Pennsylvania's is the only one that has a dissertation requirement. Other social work programs considering or planning to offer the DSW as a practice doctorate will need to determine whether to require a formal dissertation. Based on the results of this evaluation, the dissertation met the goals of contributing to the social work knowledge base and positioning DSW alumni as clinical content experts. Moreover, alumni reported that it helped them to become better scholarly writers and evidence-based practitioners. It is important to note, however, that the dissertation process requires substantial faculty resources and institutional structure and support. Programs considering the DSW would be well served to carefully take into account whether they have sufficient resources to provide the intensive mentoring and support that students need to produce high-quality dissertations in a timely manner.

In general, our experience has been that the DSW program is resource heavy and expensive to run well—with respect to both cost and labor. To maintain program quality, the school's administration has dedicated substantial fiscal, faculty, and staff resources, including staffing the program with a full-time administrative coordinator and a faculty director, providing financial incentives to standing faculty who serve on DSW dissertations, and deploying faculty to teach courses and serve on a DSW faculty governance committee. In the interest of providing the best possible educational experience, with adequate mentoring and support, we also have limited the number of entering students to 15 per year and are committed to continuing to fund renowned visiting faculty travel to campus to teach and serve on committees.

In conclusion, although the results of this evaluation of the University of Pennsylvania's program are encouraging, we are reporting on only one program with a limited number of graduates. As this program graduates more students, and other DSW programs come on line with graduates, the profession will have a better sense of whether these initial outcomes will continue or dissipate the findings reported here. It is still early in the development of this innovation for any formal conclusions to be drawn. Much remains to be learned.

## REFERENCES

Anastas, J. W. (2012). *Doctoral education in social work*. New York: Oxford University Press.

Anastas, J., & Videka, L. (2012). Does social work need a "Practice Doctorate"? *Clinical Social Work Journal, 40*, 268–276. doi:10.1007/s10615-012-0392-3

Austin, D. M. (1997). The institutional development of social work education: The first 100 years—And beyond. *Journal of Social Work Education, 33*, 599–612.

Bollag, B. (2007). Credential creep. *Chronicle of Higher Education, 53*, A10–A12.

Brekke, J. S. (2012). Shaping a science of social work. *Research on Social Work Practice, 22*, 455–464. doi:10.1177/1049731512441263

Brekke, J. S., Ell, K., & Palinka, L. A. (2007). Translational science at the National Institute for Mental Health: Can social work take its rightful place? *Research on Social Work Practice, 17*, 123–133. doi:10.1177/1049731506293693

Buchholz, S. W., Budd, G. M., Courtney, M. R., Neiheisel, M. B., Hammersla, M., & Carlson, E. D. (2013). Preparing practice scholars: Teaching knowledge application in the Doctor of Nursing practice curriculum. *Journal of the American Association of Nurse Practitioners, 25*, 473–480. doi:10.1002/2327-6924.12050

Cnaan, R. A., Draine, J., & Dichter, M. E. (2008). Introduction: An overview of the journey. In R. A. Cnaan, M. Dichter, & J. Draine (Eds.), *A century of social work and social welfare at Penn* (pp. 1–9). Philadelphia: University of Pennsylvania Press.

CSWE Commission on Accreditation. (2012). *2008 EPAS handbook*. Washington, DC: Council on Social Work Education. (Original work published 2008).

Denecke, D. D., & Frasier, H. S. (2005, November). PhD completion project: Preliminary results from baseline data. *Communicator, 38*.

Donahoe, J. N. (2000). *Advancing doctoral education in social work: The development of organizations of doctoral programs, 1948–1992* (Unpublished doctoral dissertation). University of Alabama, Tuscaloosa.

Doyle, A. (2011). History of research on process relevant to clinical social work. *Clinical Social Work Journal, 39*, 68–78. doi:10.1007/s10615-010-0296-z

Fong, R. (2012). Framing education for a science of social work. *Research on Social Work Practice, 22*, 529–536. doi:10.1177/1049731512452977

Fong, R., & Pomeroy, E. (2011). Translating research to practice. *Social Work, 56*, 5–7. doi:10.1093/sw/56.1.5

Johnson, Y. M., & Munch, S. (2010). Faculty with practice experience: The new dinosaurs in the social work academy? *Journal of Social Work Education, 46*, 57–66. doi:10.5175/JSWE.2010.200800050

Khinduka, S. (2002). Musings on doctoral education in social work. *Research on Social Work Practice, 12*, 684–694. doi:10.1177/1049731502012005007

Maxwell, T. (2003). From first to second generation professional doctorate. *Studies in Higher Education, 28*, 279–291. doi:10.1080/03075070309292

Nurius, P. S., & Kemp, S. P. (2014). Transdisciplinarity and translation: Preparing social work doctoral students for high impact research. *Research on Social Work Practice, 24*, 625–635. doi:10.1177/1049731513512375

Peterson, D. R. (1997). *Educating professional psychologists: History and guiding conception.* Washington, DC: American Psychological Association.

Pierce, D., & Peyton, C. (1999). A historical cross-disciplinary perspective on the professional doctorate in occupational therapy. *The American Journal of Occupational Therapy, 53*, 64–71. doi:10.5014/ajot.53.1.64

Reid, W. J. (1978). Some reflections on the practice doctorate. *Social Service Review, 52*, 449–455. doi:10.1086/643655

Shore, B., & Levin, A. (1991). Point/counterpoint: Is there a role for clinical doctoral social work education? No! Is there a role for clinical doctoral social work education? Yes! *Journal of Social Work Education, 27*, 231–240.

Shulman, L. S. (2010). Doctoral education shouldn't be a marathon. *Chronicle of Higher Education, 56*, B9–B12.

Shulman, L. S., Golde, C. M., Bueschel, A. C., & Garabedian, K. J. (2006). Reclaiming education's doctorates: A critique and a proposal. *Educational Researcher, 35*(3), 25–32. doi:10.3102/0013189X035003025

Social Work Policy Institute. (2013). *Advanced practice doctorates: What do they mean for social work practice, research, and education.* Washington, DC: National Association of Social Workers. Retrieved from http://www.socialwork policy.org/wp-content/uploads/2014/01/SWPI_DSW_FINAL_Report.pdf

Sowell, R. (2008). *PhD completion and attrition: Analysis of baseline data.* Washington, DC: Council of Graduate Schools.

Starck, P. L., Duffy, M. E., & Vogler, R. (1993). Developing a nursing doctorate for the 21st century. *Journal of Professional Nursing, 9*, 212–219. doi:10.1016/8755-7223(93)90038-E

Talbert, R. L. (1997). ACCP strategic planning conference: Issues and trends in clinical pharmacy education. *Pharmacotherapy: The Journal of Human Pharmacology and Drug Therapy, 17*, 1073–1078.

Task Force on the DSW Degree. (2011). *The doctorate in social work (DSW) degree: Emergence of a new practice doctorate.* Retrieved from http://www.cswe.org/CentersInitiatives/DataStatistics/ProgramData/59952.aspx

Threlkeld, A. J., Jensen, G. M., & Royeen, C. B. (1999). The clinical doctorate: A framework for analysis in physical therapist education. *Physical Therapy*, *79*, 567–581.

Thyer, B. A. (1997). Promoting research on community practice using single system research designs. In R. H. MacNair (Ed.), *Research studies in community practice* (pp. 47–61). Binghamton, NY: Haworth.

Thyer, B. A. (2002). Evidenced-based practice and clinical social work. *Evidence Based Mental Health*, *5*, 6–7.

Zastrow, C., & Bremner, J. (2004). Social work education responds to the shortage of persons with both a doctorate and a professional social work degree. *Journal of Social Work Education*, *40*, 351–358.

# Preparing Emerging Doctoral Scholars for Transdisciplinary Research: A Developmental Approach

SUSAN PATRICIA KEMP and PAULA S. NURIUS

*School of Social Work, University of Washington, Seattle, Washington, USA*

*Research models that bridge disciplinary, theoretical, and methodological boundaries are increasingly common as funders and the public push for effective responses to pressing social problems. Although social work is inherently an integrative discipline, there is growing recognition of the need to better prepare emerging scholars for sophisticated transdisciplinary and translational research environments. This article outlines a developmental, competency-oriented approach to enhancing the readiness of doctoral students and emerging scholars in social work and allied disciplines for transdisciplinary research, describes an array of pedagogical tools applicable in doctoral course work, and urges coordinated attention to enhancing the field's transdisciplinary training capacity.*

Transdisciplinarity has been described as "research across disciplinary boundaries and in collaboration with stakeholders . . . [that] orients scientific research towards issues of social concern" (Tötzer, Sedlacek, & Knoflacher, 2011, pp. 840–841). A primary driver of transdisciplinary (TD) research is the need for timely and innovative responses to complex real-world issues. Calls for collaborative, impact-oriented science resonate with social work, which has always been concerned with linking its science, service, and social change missions (Kirk & Reid, 2002). As an integrative, boundary-spanning profession (Mor Barak & Brekke, 2014; Oliver, 2013), social work is well positioned for leadership in TD efforts. An emphasis on cross-disciplinary research therefore has emerged in discussions regarding shaping a science of social work (Brekke, 2012, 2013).

Proposals to focus the profession on meeting grand challenges (Grand Challenges Executive Committee, 2014), as well as the Society for Social Work & Research 2012–2017 strategic plan, and the Group for the Advancement of Doctoral Education in Social Work *Quality Guidelines for Doctoral Education* (Harrington, Petr, Black, Cunningham-Williams, & Bentley, 2013) all are responsive to this trend. As public health scholars have noted, "A radical shift toward greater integration among disciplines and greater integration between knowledge production and its application, calls for similar educational transformation" (Neuhauser, Richardson, Mackenzie, & Minkler, 2007, p. 10).

Sarah Gehlert (2012; Gehlert & Browne, 2013) has strongly advocated a pipeline approach to TD education, beginning in doctoral programs and building toward postdoctoral and early career training opportunities. In sustainability science, where TD research is well established, attention is likewise shifting from short-term training modalities to longer term educational strategies (Lyall & Meagher, 2012). Similar calls are evident in public health (Krettek & Thorpenberg, 2011; Larson, Landers, & Begg, 2011; Neuhauser et al., 2007) and social ecology (Stokols, 2014).

Given the emergent nature of these discussions, the literature on the practicality of preparing doctoral students for TD research is still relatively modest. Helpful guidance is afforded by the work of Stokols and his colleagues in the School of Social Ecology at the University of California Irvine (Misra, Stokols, Hall, & Feng, 2011; Stokols, 2014), by various publications based on experiences with National Science Foundation–funded Integrative Graduate Education and Research Traineeships (IGERTs; Graybill et al., 2006; Graybill & Shandas, 2010; Schmidt et al., 2012), by scholars of higher education (Manathunga, Lant, & Mellick, 2006), and via publications and training materials produced by several groups outside the United States, primarily in sustainability science (Lyall & Meagher, 2012, Mitchell, 2009). In social work, useful framing materials can be found in Gehlert's publications (Gehlert, 2012; Gehlert & Browne, 2013) and in materials related to discussions of social work and science (e.g., Davis, 2011; Fong, 2012, 2013; Kemp & Nurius, 2013; Mor Barak & Brekke, 2014; Nurius & Kemp, 2013, 2014). In general, however, these resources stop short of offering specific curricular or programmatic suggestions.

With the goal of moving these discussions a step closer to the realities of doctoral education, this article outlines a framework for enhancing TD readiness in social work doctoral programs and is illustrated by practical and pedagogical tools applicable to coursework and other program components. We recognize that social work doctoral programs already expose their students to a variety of cross-disciplinary learning experiences. Nevertheless, we see additional opportunities for crafting an approach to TD development that builds on and amplifies learning opportunities already in place, creates new ones as appropriate, and more intentionally scaffolds the learning process for doctoral students.

The material presented is based on work that the authors have been doing in their own doctoral program, as well as a thorough assessment of the available literature and related materials in other fields. It also is informed by our experiences spanning very different kinds of interdisciplinary and transdisciplinary research efforts. Susan Kemp's scholarship entails broad-based collaboration with colleagues in the spatial sciences and design professions, including geography, architecture, urban planning, and landscape design, as well an orientation to public health and environmental science. In contrast, Paula Nurius's work focuses on multilevel models relating to health and development outcomes and disparities, drawing from multiple health and social science disciplines that operationalize mechanisms through which the effects of environmental adversity are conveyed and life course stress is biologically embodied. Common to both experiences is a recognition that transdisciplinary expertise is hard come by, even for social work scholars with strong grounding in relational practice.

To ground the article in a common language, we provide brief definitions of disciplinary terminology. We then outline and elaborate on a developmental approach, grounded in core TD competencies and attributes, aimed at enhancing the readiness of social work doctoral students for TD research. Because we view preparation for TD research as equally (if differentially) important for students in the practice doctorates, who are particularly well positioned for collaborative, boundary-spanning practice-based research (Anastas & Videka, 2012), our aim is to chart a road map broadly germane to doctoral training in social work. Individual programs can then determine the best fit, relative to their training priorities and the characteristics of their educational and community setting.

## DEFINING DISCIPLINARY RELATIONSHIPS

The terms *unidisciplinary, multidisciplinary, interdisciplinary,* and *transdisciplinary* share points of overlap but also represent differing configurations and implications. Viewed broadly, they represent a continuum of increasing disciplinary integration and interdependence. Each can be pursued by a single scholar or by teams working together on a particular research enterprise. We use the umbrella term *cross-disciplinary* when referring to discipline-spanning models overall. The following definitions build from those suggested by Gehlert et al. (2008), Hall (2013), Nash (2008), Rosenfield (1992), and Stokols (2006) and include examples of related programmatic components.

## Unidisciplinary (UD)

Scholars from a single discipline work together within a common, discipline-defined framework. Drawing on the "apples and oranges" metaphor, Hall (2013) represents unidisciplinarity as a single type of fruit. Disciplines are defined by their histories, priorities, and definitional boundaries as well as their conceptual and methodological tools and lenses. Socialization to a discipline is an important part of doctoral training, often pursued through cohort-based coursework involving only (or predominantly) students within a discipline or program, with content attentive to the discipline's history, central tenets, and commitments. Program requirements (e.g., the general examination, dissertation) often involve articulation and defense of a plan of study relative to a home discipline's values and priorities.

## Multidisciplinary (MD)

Scholars from different disciplines work together, separately or sequentially, on common research questions or goals but maintain their primary disciplinary frameworks (visualize a platter with a variety of different fruits on it). Students may achieve some degree of multidisciplinary training through courses taken in other departments. Many times these "outside" courses are anchored in another home discipline (e.g., psychology, sociology), providing students with valuable information about that discipline's knowledge, methods, and perspectives. Varying degrees of integration can evolve through this type of exposure, but that outcome is not assured. Unless classrooms are constructed to stimulate purposeful interactions among students, or assignments press for integrative outcomes, students tend to exit doctoral education with multidiscipline breadth but limited synthesis.

## Interdisciplinary (ID)

Scholars work jointly on a common problem with the intention of transferring knowledge from one discipline to another; hence, ID collaborations are marked by researchers regularly interacting with and influencing one another. ID-oriented courses tend to emphasize the interrelationships among disciplinary perspectives. Courses and programs may require students to articulate an integrated distillation of content, theory, or methodologies that prompts multidomain or multilevel understanding. Theoretical and methodological training typically allows a deeper grasp of findings and connections across disciplinary divides. Metaphorically, ID training may be represented as a fruit salad: Through the training process, students craft linkages across disciplines while retaining their individual disciplinary identities. Frequently, students are also encouraged to hone skills that facilitate communication, comprehension, and innovation across disciplinary borders.

## Transdisciplinary (TD)

Scholars work collaboratively to transfer knowledge and methods, develop shared conceptual frameworks, and generate novel methodologies. Extending the fruit metaphor, TD teams can be thought of as "smoothies"—each participant works at the interface of the collective disciplines to more fully grasp complex causal mechanisms and craft novel and accelerated solutions. A TD orientation is typically multilevel (e.g., cells to societies) (Gehlert et al., 2008), attentive to complex relationships among mechanisms, and methodologically pluralistic (Cassinari et al., 2011, Stokols, 2006). Increasingly, transdisciplinarity involves close collaboration between researchers and community stakeholders, who work together to understand and ultimately resolve collectively identified problems (Cram & Phillips, 2012).

## TRANSDISCIPLINARY READINESS: CORE DOMAINS AND COMPETENCIES

Effective participation in TD research calls for disciplinary depth, the ability to both navigate and integrate diverse methodological and theoretical frameworks, and sophisticated communication and collaborative skills. Klein (2004) described transdisciplinarity as "simultaneously an attitude and an action" (p. 521). Transdisciplinary scholars tend to be "inclusive . . . thinkers, broad gauged and contextually oriented in their theorizing and research, methodologically eclectic, . . . open-minded and respectful of divergent view points, and adept at promoting good will and cross-discipline tolerance" (Mitrany & Stokols, 2005, p. 439). Although social work students typically enter doctoral education with strong relational skills, additional training may be needed to hone the research integration skills central to confident participation in TD scholarship. These metacognitive, scientific, and collaborative skills are summarized in Table 1.

The competencies in Table 1 provide a valuable point of reference in considering how best to programmatically enhance TD readiness. At Washington University's Brown School, for example, faculty in the public health program constructed a set of learning experiences (and related outcome competencies) regarding students' ability to *explain* why complex problems benefit from TD approaches; to *describe, distinguish, develop*, and *apply* theories, methods, and TD competencies in problem solving research; and to *communicate* TD evidence to stakeholders with the aim of influencing policy and practice (Arnold, Kuhlmann, Hipp, & Budd, 2013). This form of competency-oriented thinking provides a helpful model for mapping where and how to incorporate TD-oriented content within and across courses and other program elements.

**TABLE 1** Transdisciplinary Readiness: Qualities and Competencies

By the end of their doctoral programs, students will be able to:

**Critically Engage, Reflect, and Integrate:**
Demonstrate critical awareness of the underlying assumptions of their own discipline, its scope, contributions, and limitations
Navigate and reflexively engage multiple disciplinary languages, perspectives, and worldviews
Think broadly and contextually about complex, multilevel problems
Identify higher order relationships, synthesize, and integrate

**Collaborate:**
Engage colleagues from other disciplines and community stakeholders to gain their perspectives on research problems, frameworks, or topics
Respect the roles and contributions of others
Effectively navigate tensions and conflict
Stay at the table (persistence)

**Communicate:**
Explain their own work and perspectives clearly and confidently to others
Read publications and attend conferences beyond her or his own discipline
Disseminate research results within and beyond her or his own discipline
Publish with colleagues from other disciplines

**Conduct Research:**
Flexibly use theories from multiple disciplines in developing integrative, multilevel conceptual frameworks
Integrate concepts and methods from multiple disciplines in designing research protocols
Modify research agenda as a result of interactions and input from other colleagues
Design, seek funding for, and implement interdisciplinary research projects in collaboration with scholars from other disciplines and community stakeholders.

*Note.* Adapted from Gebbie et al. (2008), Hall (2013), Larson et al. (2011), Nash (2008), and Stokols (2014).

## CULTIVATING TRANSDISCIPLINARY READINESS: A SCAFFOLDED DEVELOPMENTAL APPROACH

The approach to TD preparation detailed next rests on two interlocking assumptions. First, we take a developmental approach, keeping in mind students' maturational trajectories as emerging scholars, the incremental nature of doctoral education, and the importance of appropriately aligning TD learning with both these realities. One likely would think differently, for example, about TD preparation for 1st-year students than for those who are writing dissertations and preparing to graduate. Drawing from Graybill et al. (2006) and Graybill and Shandas (2010), we conceptualize this developmental trajectory as beginning with *initiation*, progressing to *navigation*, and concluding with *maturation* (see Figure 1). Although for heuristic purposes we present this progression as linear, we are acutely aware that learning is recursive and that in reality no hard lines can be drawn between one point in students' TD development and another.

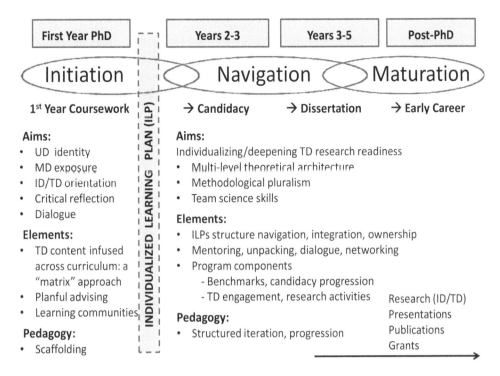

**FIGURE 1** Transdisciplinary (TD) developmental road map.

In addition, supporting students' maturation as transdisciplinary and translational scholars requires careful institutional, pedagogical, and interpersonal scaffolding, not only through coursework but in other key elements of doctoral education, including research experiences, mentoring, advising, and dialogue with peers. Most social work doctoral programs actively encourage students to take courses in other departments, but often it is left to the students to process and make sense out of these learning experiences. In Anastas's (2012) recent survey of social work doctoral programs, respondents noted this reality as often problematic, leading to confusion, reticence, and even outright reluctance to continue pursuing cross-disciplinary training opportunities. The literature on TD development, in contrast, emphasizes the importance of providing students with consistent, ongoing structural supports, threaded throughout their training (Graybill et al., 2006). Because the influences on students' scholarly development are both multiple and cumulative, such curricular scaffolding needs to be thoughtfully staged to provide iterative opportunities for developing and consolidating the core TD competencies outlined in Table 1. The following principles, derived from the TD literature, provide general guidance:

1. *Begin early*: There is increasing concurrence that preparation for ID/TD research should begin early and be threaded iteratively throughout

students' training (Gehlert, 2012; Stokols, 2014). Recognizing that this approach raises concerns about the potential dilution of students' disciplinary identities as social work scholars—and that disciplinary depth is an essential prerequisite for effective transdisciplinarity—we view ID/TD preparation as complementary to (rather than a replacement for) disciplinary preparation.

2. *Mix and phase forms of disciplinary training and exposure*: Klein (2008) pointed out that educational benefits derive from each aspect of disciplinarity and from "quadrangulation," or purposeful gleaning from the strengths of each—gaining, for example, depth from UD, breadth from MD, integration from ID, and competencies for new forms of team science from TD. Just as forms of disciplinarity represent a continuum from less to more integrative, so will emphases vary across students' programs of study—typically moving from an initial focus on UD training to a deepening concentration on cross-disciplinary engagement and synthesis (Misra et al., 2011).

3. *Infuse TD content throughout courses and program elements*: Ideally, TD coursework and related learning experiences are threaded both horizontally and vertically throughout the curriculum. An excellent example of a "matrix" approach to TD training can be found in Neuhauser et al.'s (2007) description of the development of a TD doctoral program in public health. This approach contrasts with tendencies to either rely on the broad theoretical and methodological overviews provided in foundational survey courses or bracket TD content in later electives (Pallas, 2001).

4. *Incorporate a mix of didactic and experiential teaching methods and learning experiences*: Given that TD competence blends relational, communicative, conceptual, and methodological skills, multiple pedagogical approaches are required to support students' TD development (Frodeman, Klein, Mitcham, & Holbrook, 2010). Active, experiential, team-based learning therefore is essential: "Through collaboration . . . students develop critical thinking skills that help them understand the value of others' perspectives, tolerate ambiguity in problem-solving situations, establish productive habits of communication. . . , and build interdependent working relationships" (Wagner, Baum, & Newbill, 2013, p. 1).

5. *Provide opportunities for shared dialogue and reflection*: Learning communities emerge in the literature as critical to mutual support, intellectual exchange, and identity formation (Mor Barak & Brekke, 2014; Willetts & Mitchell, 2006). TD learning is facilitated when students have structured opportunities for dialogue with each other and more senior colleagues around difficult questions related to integration, bridging cross-disciplinary differences, and the development of "habit[s] of responsible participation" (Klein, 2014, p. 26). Reflecting on their experiences in an IGERT training program, by way of illustration, Graybill et al. (2006)

pointed to the central importance of expertly facilitated opportunities to process often complex learning experiences.

## INITIATION: THE 1ST-YEAR DOCTORAL CURRICULUM

The 1st year of social work doctoral education typically focuses on two elements: (a) orienting incoming students to their new roles as social work scholars, and (b) providing them with a strong theoretical, methodological, and policy foundation for later individualized programs of study. Appropriately, required courses and related learning opportunities foreshadow disciplinary (UD) socialization (see Figure 1). Nonetheless, this 1st year also affords important opportunities to expose students to the landscape of ID/TD research and lay an initial base for the development of a TD orientation. Consistent with the matrix approach just described, such orienting content ideally will be distributed across 1st-year coursework, with required courses incorporating those elements most relevant to students' particular foci and aims. Methods courses, for example, may include readings and discussions orienting students to developments in translational and TD research and related competencies. Social policy courses may underscore the ways in which policy knowledge and research inform multilevel approaches to pressing social issues. Theory courses, including those focused primarily on social science theory, provide necessary foundations to diverse scholarly traditions.

Often underemphasized, however, are opportunities for developing the epistemological skills foundational to supple engagement with diverse theoretical and methodological frameworks. As suggested in Table 1, these competencies include students' ability to demonstrate critical awareness of the underlying assumptions of their own discipline, its scope, contributions, and limitations, and to navigate and reflexively engage multiple disciplinary languages, worldviews, theories, and methods.

Courses that include the philosophy of social science or exploration of different theoretical and methodological paradigms are particularly appropriate venues for a sharpened focus on these skill sets. Pedagogical elements that support such development include the following:

1. Structured opportunities for students to reflect on their personal knowledge frameworks.
2. Course content that not only immerses students in core disciplinary frameworks but also allows for critical reflection on disciplinary assumptions.
3. Readings, presentations (e.g., guest speakers from other disciplines), and discussions that expose students to contrasting knowledge paradigms and disciplinary worldviews, preparing them to "understand, appreciate, and

assimilate the alterative philosophical assumptions, constructs, and methods associated with disparate fields and levels of analysis" (Stokols, 2014, p. 71)

4. Conversation and dialogue with peers, within and beyond the students' home discipline, aimed at strengthening communication and collaboration skills.

To illustrate potential teaching strategies, we offer two brief examples, the first from the lead author's doctoral theory course, and the second developed in a National Science Foundation–funded IGERT project (Eigenbrode et al., 2007).

## INTELLECTUAL BIOGRAPHIES

Students come to doctoral education with worldviews and intellectual frameworks already deeply shaped by their personal, cultural, educational, and professional experiences. Those with social work degrees (and related practice experience) may have to make an often challenging shift in identity from practitioner to scholar (Mor Barak & Brekke, 2014). A simple strategy for stimulating reflection on and conversation about the assumptions students bring with them is to elicit students' intellectual biographies: the personal, cultural, and educational experiences that inform their current intellectual and conceptual frameworks. We have found that sharing intellectual biographies (including the instructor's) in the first session of our 1st-year theory course underscores the diverse intellectual resources in the class, increases students' awareness of their own and others' training and disciplinary assumptions, and serves as a useful point of reference when the course content explores different knowledge paradigms. This orientation to one another's intellectual frameworks also gives students and instructors ways of interpreting and understanding each other beyond identity markers such as gender, race, age, ethnicity, or sexual orientation.

### The Toolbox Dialogue Method

The Toolbox is a structured method for facilitating individual reflection and collective dialogue regarding the fundamental conceptual, methodological, and value assumptions underlying differences in approaches to research. Frequently left unexplored, these assumptions are highly consequential—and often problematic—in the context of collaborative research. Grounded in philosophy, the Toolbox facilitates the identification and exploration of epistemological differences, whether by an individual student or in a group. Developed in the context of science–technology–engineering–medicine research (Eigenbrode et al., 2007), it also has been adapted for translational behavioral research (Schnapp et al., 2012). Organized around a set of core questions, the Toolbox questionnaire is a useful, relatively straightforward method for generating discussion about issues that frequently underlie misunderstandings not only in research teams but among students in doctoral seminar discussions. Illustrative core questions include the following: What is your primary motivation for conducting research? Do values have a legitimate role in research? What types of evidentiary support are required for knowledge? Must scientific research be objective to be legitimate (Eigenbrode et al., 2007; Schnapp ct al., 2012)?

## Involving Students From Other Disciplines

We have found that discussions such as these frequently are richer and more productive when they include students from other disciplines. Many social work doctoral programs have a tradition of cohort-based approaches to the 1st year of doctoral coursework. Although discipline-centric content and identity formation are clearly important, our experience has been that involving students from other doctoral programs in social work courses does not threaten the disciplinary identities of social work doctoral students. Rather, sister discipline involvement enriches discussions, providing opportunities for students to share different perspectives and examine one another's assumptions. Cross-disciplinary exploration and exchanges conducted *within* a social work frame of reference also orient students from other disciplines to the nature and contributions of social work research. We therefore are enthusiastic about the potential for more proactively opening up social work doctoral courses, for example, by reworking and "rebranding" existing courses so that they attract doctoral students from programs beyond social work.

## Advising and Mentoring

First-year advisors play a key role in assisting students to navigate and make connections across their various learning experiences, serving as a sounding board as students begin to think through their programs of study beyond the required foundational coursework, brokering connections for students with colleagues in other disciplines, and reviewing external courses and research opportunities. The emphasis here is on advising that is planned and anticipatory. Clearly, TD learning should be appropriately tailored to students' educational development and research aims. Nonetheless, graduates reflecting back on their training experiences emphasize the critical role of early and ongoing planning to later TD readiness (Graybill et al., 2006).

## BEYOND INITIATION: DEVELOPMENTAL NAVIGATION AND MATURATION

By the end of the 1st year, doctoral students are moving beyond prescribed foundation coursework and beginning to construct individualized programs of study oriented to their own areas of focus and specialization. In this section, we describe a range of planning, instructional, and mentoring tools relevant to scaffolding students' ongoing TD development.

### Individualized Learning Plans (ILPs)

ILPs (sometimes referred to as Individual Development Plans) provide a structure wherein students frame initial statements of their research aims and then iteratively hone these as they progress through a variety of learning experiences (e.g., coursework, independent studies, qualifying examinations, research assistant opportunities, dissertations).[1] ILPs serve a range of helpful functions in relation to TD development, particularly around planning and coherence. As scaffolding tools, they encourage students to justify their selection of theoretical, substantive, and research methods courses and the cross-disciplinary linkages that appear most important to their research goals. These selections, in turn, form an individualized foundation for the incremental development of more fully integrated theoretical models, methodological tools appropriate to students' aims, and the collaborative skills needed to function effectively in research teams in their substantive arena.

### Transdisciplinary Seminars

It is not typical for social work doctoral programs to construct courses specifically designed to attract graduate students from across campus and, thereby, create incubators for ID and TD engagement and integration. In our experience, however, such courses provide a number of important benefits: (a) increased recognition of social work's value as a campus resource for (and not only consumer of) doctoral-level courses; (b) opportunities for social work faculty to forefront disciplinary priorities, such as reducing disparities and optimizing health-promoting environments; and (c) integrative occasions for engaging with colleagues from multiple disciplines—both student and faculty—around a social or health topic of shared interest. (For illustrations

---

[1]    Examples of individualized learning plan guidelines and formats can be found at the Intersections of Mental Health Perspectives in Addictions Research Training (http://www.addiction sresearchtraining.ca/resources/forms.html) and the University of Washington social work doctoral program (http://socialwork.uw.edu/programs/phd-manuals-forms/guidelines-for-the-program-of-study-leading-to-the-general-examination-0).

of curricula and course structures designed to foster a TD orientation, including pipeline considerations from undergraduate through postgraduate, see Larson et al., 2011; Lyall & Meagher, 2012; and Stokols, 2014.)

We have been part of TD-oriented courses focused on prevention science, stress embodiment, health disparities, and people–place relationships, each of which has included differing disciplinary sets of students. As a result, pedagogical elements that we have found useful in furthering ID/TD goals include the following:

1. Explicit framing in the course description and goals regarding disciplinary integration across the course content and among the participating students.
2. Structuring the course curriculum to illuminate both specialized disciplinary contributions (e.g., neuroendocrinology of stress) and interdisciplinary applications or integration (e.g., integration of neurophysiology into frameworks that account for environmental factors, lifespan development, psychological mediators, and tools usable by nonbiological specialists).
3. Inclusion of faculty from other disciplines to illustrate theories and methods distinctive to their discipline but germane to the course focus (with the core instructor ensuring integrative coherence of content).
4. Activities that foster students' cross-disciplinary interaction (e.g., identifying disciplinary lenses, eliciting succinct cross-disciplinary consultation on one another's models, spontaneous construction of hypothetical collaborations among small, mixed disciplinary groups), scaffolded by guidelines for communication and navigation of differences.
5. Course assignments that require each student to produce an ID/TD product appropriate to the course goals and the student's level of training (e.g., an abbreviated, mock grant proposal; a briefing document describing a new TD-oriented researcher role, or research team needed to investigate the student's research topic; a neighborhood assessment representing integrative multidisciplinary perspectives).

Transdisciplinary courses such as these provide rich opportunities for fostering and deepening many of the qualities and competencies identified in Table 1. We have found that students often use such course assignments to help develop their thinking toward qualifying examinations, dissertations, or grant proposals—such as drawing multilevel "box and arrow" theoretical models, with summaries designed to be understandable to colleagues in other disciplines, as well as stakeholders in the field. Guided opportunities designed to strengthen students' abilities to communicate effectively in these venues serve as powerful aids in solidifying the "cognitive architecture" underpinning their theoretical perspectives, as well as their confidence, as social welfare researchers, now conversant in a larger platform of science.

## Matrix Planning Across Program Components

As students move into the more individualized parts of their doctoral training, they need structured opportunities to progressively turn their intellectual fruit platters into fruit salads—and ultimately (even if post-PhD) into smoothie-style syntheses. Program elements, such as general examinations, the dissertation prospectus, and research activities, are key platforms for the development of integrative ID and TD research readiness. Incorporating TD-focused aims into these core program components provides students and their mentoring faculty with benchmarks that also can be included in their ILPs. Building on coursework, these program components are important pedagogical vehicles for the navigation and maturation phases (see Figure 1), wherein students progressively refine their own intellectual architecture, deepen their team science readiness, and begin to develop some of the more advanced competencies outlined in Table 1. Meaningful achievement of these goals in the more individualized phases of doctoral education is enhanced significantly by clear guidelines (e.g., in program benchmarks for completion, advising checklists) and TD-oriented mentoring and supervision.

## Evolving Mentoring Considerations

As noted, students need ongoing opportunities to connect the dots across these various experiences. Ideally, students will have a consistent relationship over time with a primary mentor who works with the student to develop and actualize her or his individualized learning plan. Increasingly, ID/TD-oriented supervision may also involve multiple mentors with expertise spanning disciplines or specializations. Key mentoring roles include helping students involved in cross-disciplinary training to stay focused on their particular ID/TD goals and to set boundaries that appropriately balance depth, breadth, and complexity (Graybill et al., 2006). Issues of scope and balance are salient across TD training, from course selection and qualifying examinations to decisions about hybrid dissertations and collaborative publications.

Supporting students in tolerating and persisting through the ambiguity inherent in constructing a synthesized research identity, and operating in the spaces between disciplines, is essential (Wagner et al., 2013). One place where tension often manifests is in ID doctoral committees, which require both students and mentors to engage with "unfamiliar others" who bring differences in disciplinary and departmental languages, methodologies, and cultures (Fuqua, Stokols, Gress, Phillips, & Harvey, 2004; Nash, 2008). Traditionally, such committees have tended to function in a multidisciplinary fashion, with members from other disciplines providing their expertise and looking for ways that this expertise is well represented in the student's work. As Olivero (2014) pointed out, this classical model is not well suited to a more explicitly integrationist agenda. Lyall and Meagher (2012) illustrated conundrums that may evolve, such as committee members expecting chapters targeted to their respective disciplinary interests, or only being willing to review elements familiar to their discipline. To support students' TD development, lead mentors and program directors will need to foster changes in supervisory committee norms—for example, to encourage integrated rather than compartmentalized products, or publications accessible to readers spanning relevant disciplines and stakeholders.

## MENTORING IN RESEARCH TRAINING

Research activities should come more centrally under the umbrella of mentoring. Many social work research teams are multidisciplinary, yet research practica and assistantships tend to focus on training students in research methods and miss opportunities to make visible to students the processes underlying ID/TD research. For example, how did they arrive at an integrated theoretical formulation? Or negotiate conflicting perspectives within the team about how best to operationalize mechanisms spanning levels of phenomena? This kind of modeling provides students with "how to" insights vital to successfully navigating real-world ID/TD research collaborations upon graduation.

The qualities that make for effective ID/TD mentors overlap those needed in students, such as open-mindedness; curiosity toward learning from other disciplines; and willingness to undertake challenges such as mastering new languages, questioning disciplinary assumptions, navigating tensions that come with differences, along with focus and persistence. Lyall, Meagher, and Tait (2008) noted appropriately that TD-oriented students often test out a range of disciplinary frameworks before settling on the right mix. Mentoring these students involves serving as a thoughtful sounding board, as well as being able to explicate the practicalities associated with facilitating cross-disciplinary connections while maintaining steady progress. Helpful guidelines for TD mentoring have been developed by the Institute for the Study of Science Technology and Innovation (see ISSTI, 2014).

## GROUP MENTORING

Group mentoring models also hold promise, with one or a small group of faculty taking the lead, working closely with the doctoral program director, and exchanging resources and feedback on experiences with instructional and mentoring faculty. For example, we have found considerable value in seminars that purposefully engage students across multiple years within our program as well as students from other disciplines (Mech, 2001). To foster a sense of trust within a collegial learning community, these yearlong seminars have expectations of regular participation. We have drawn from a number of resources in structuring scenarios and engagement activities (see, e.g., ISSTI, n.d.; Lyall, Bruce, Tait, & Meagher, 2011; Mitchell, 2009; Team Science Toolkit [https://www.teamsciencetoolkit.cancer.gov/public/home.aspx?js=1])

## BEYOND THE PHD

Evaluations of transdisciplinary doctoral programs (Mitrany & Stokols, 2005) suggest that by the time they graduate, participating students will have developed a strong ID orientation and a platform of readiness for entering ID/TD research careers. To be fully successful in TD research team relationships, roles, and productivity, early career graduates nonetheless will need continued mentoring and institutional scaffolding. As students prepare to graduate, they therefore will need to be charting the postgraduation steps of their TD road map with mentors, reflecting on what they need to look for in their next scholarly environment, and planning the strategic development of scholarly portfolios, which illustrate expertise in their home discipline, as well as a readiness to engage with other disciplines in research design, implementation, and translation (Hall et al., 2012; Millar, 2013).

## CONCLUDING NOTE

At the 2014 Society for Social Work and Research annual conference, a roundtable session on the science of social work fostered a productive conversation about issues related to promoting social work's capacity to excel as an integrative scientific discipline. To our perception, it was doctoral students and early career faculty who most clearly reflected a sense of urgency about crafting and sustaining such a productive research career in contemporary research environments. The issues they raised were specific, pragmatic, and real-time; for them, the moment for capacity building is now. Discussions in a workshop at the same conference had a similar flavor. The doctoral students in particular were both immersed in cross-disciplinary experiences and eager for more programmatic support and guidance. Although there are few off-the-shelf, one-size-fits-all solutions, other fields and sister disciplines offer useful tools and experiences. Drawing on these, we have attempted in this article to outline a pragmatic approach to strengthening social work's transdisciplinary doctoral training capacity by building on existing program elements while leaving room for programmatic diversity. We encourage social work doctoral programs to experiment; a good deal can be achieved by amplifying areas of existing readiness and crafting stronger and more explicit connections. But there is also room for boldness—for social work doctoral education to mirror, in fact, the spirit of urgency, innovation, and openness to change that animates the best of transdisciplinary science.

# REFERENCES

Anastas, J. (2012). *Doctoral education in social work*. New York, NY: Oxford University Press.

Anastas, J., & Videka, L. (2012). Does social work need a "practice doctorate"? *Clinical Social Work Journal*, *40*, 268–276. doi:10.1007/s10615-012-0392-3

Arnold, L. D., Kuhlmann, A. S., Hipp, J. A., & Budd, E. (2013). Competencies in transdisciplinary public health education. In D. Haire-Joshu & T. D. McBride (Eds.), *Transdisciplinary public health: Research, education, and practice* (pp. 53–76). San Francisco, CA: Jossey Bass.

Brekke, J. S. (2012). Shaping a science of social work. *Research on Social Work Practice*, *22*, 455–464. doi:10.1177/1049731512441263

Brekke, J. S. (2013). A science of social work, and social work as an integrative scientific discipline: Have we gone too far, or not far enough? *Research on Social Work Practice*. Advance online publication. doi:1049731513511994

Cassinari, D., Hillier, J., Miciukiewicz, K., Novy, A., Habersack, K., MacCallum, D., & Moulaert, F. (2011). *Transdisciplinary research in social polis*. Retrieved from https://lirias.kuleuven.be/bitstream/123456789/339693/1/Trans_final_web_single_page.pdf

Cram, F., & Phillips, H. (2012). Claiming interstitial space for multicultural, transdisciplinary research through community-up values. *International Journal of Critical Indigenous Studies*, *5*, 36–49.

Davis, K. (2011, January). *The youngest science: Social work research as product and process in a competitive scientific market*. Invited presidential address, Society for Social Work & Research, Tampa, FL.

Eigenbrode, S. D., O'Rourke, M., Wulfhorst, J. D., Althoff, D. M., Goldberg, C. S., Merrill, K., . . . Bosque-Pérez, N. A. (2007). Employing philosophical dialogue in collaborative science. *BioScience*, *57*, 55–64. doi:10.1641/B570109

Fong, R. (2012). Framing education for a science of social work: Missions, curriculum, and doctoral training. *Research on Social Work Practice*, *22*, 529–536. doi:10.1177/1049731512452977

Fong, R. (2013). Framing doctoral education for a science of social work: Positioning students for the scientific career, promoting scholars for the academy, propagating scientists of the profession, and preparing stewards of the discipline. *Research on Social Work Practice*. Advance online publication. doi:10.1177/1049731513515055

Frodeman, R., Klein, J. T., Mitcham, C., & Holbrook, J. B. (2010). *The Oxford handbook of interdisciplinarity*. Oxford, UK: Oxford University Press.

Fuqua, J., Stokols, D., Gress, J., Phillips, K., & Harvey, R. (2004). Transdisciplinary collaboration as a basis for enhancing the science and prevention of substance use and "abuse." *Substance Use & Misuse*, *39*, 1457–1514. doi:10.1081/JA-200033200

Gebbie, K. M., Meier, B. M., Bakken, S., Carrasquillo, O., Formicola, A., Aboelela, S. W., . . . Larson, E. (2008). Training for interdisciplinary health research: Defining the required competencies. *Journal of Allied Health*, *37*(2), 65–70.

Gehlert, S. (2012). Shaping education and training to advance transdisciplinary health research. *Transdisciplinary Journal of Engineering and Science*, *3*, 1–10.

Gehlert, S., & Browne, T. (2013). Transdisciplinary training and education. In D. Haire-Joshu & T. D. McBride (Eds.), *Transdisciplinary public health: Research, education, and practice* (pp. 31–51). San Francisco, CA: Jossey-Bass.

Gehlert, S., Sohmer, D., Sacks, T., Mininger, C., McClintock, M., & Olopade, O. (2008). Targeting health disparities. A model linking upstream determinants to downstream interventions. *Health Affairs, 27,* 339–349. doi:10.1377/hlthaff.27.2.339

Grand Challenges Executive Committee. (2014). Grand challenges for social work. *Journal of the Society for Social Work and Research, 4,* 165–170. doi:10.5243/jsswr.2013.11

Graybill, J. K., Dooling, S., Shandas, V., Withey, J., Greve, A., & Simon, G. L. (2006). A rough guide to interdisciplinarity: Graduate student perspectives. *BioScience, 56,* 757–763. doi:10.1641/0006-3568(2006)56[757:ARGTIG]2.0.CO;2

Graybill, J. K., & Shandas, V. (2010). Doctoral student and early career academic perspectives. In R. Frodeman, J. T. Klein, & C. Mitcham (Eds.), *The Oxford handbook of interdisciplinarity* (pp. 404–418). New York, NY: Oxford University Press.

Hall, K. L. (2013, April). *Transdisciplinary research: Conceptual and practical issues.* Paper presented at the Transdisciplinary Translation for Prevention of High Risk Behaviors Conference. Retrieved from http://www.ttpr.org/images/2013_Presentation/_Keynote_Hall_2013.pdf

Hall, K. L., Vogel, A. L., Stipelman, B. A., Stokols, D., Morgan, G., & Gehlert, S. (2012). A four-phase model of transdisciplinary team-based research: Goals, team processes, and strategies. *Translational Behavioral Methods, 2*(4), 1–16.

Harrington, D., Petr, C., Black, M., Cunningham-Williams, R. M., & Bentley, K. J. (2013). Quality guidelines for social work PhD programs. *Research on Social Work Practice.* Advance online publication. doi:10.1177/1049731513517145

Institute for the Study of Science Technology and Innovation. (2014) Briefing notes series. Retrieved from http://www.issti.ed.ac.uk/resources/briefing_notes

Institute for the Study of Science Technology and Innovation. (n.d.). *Interdisciplinary Wiki Homepage.* Retrieved from https://www.wiki.ed.ac.uk/display/ISSTIInterdisciplinary/Interdisciplinary+Wiki+Homepage;jsessionid=2CAF39E37B77B60536CB2BE0DB7F4133

Kemp, S. P., & Nurius, P. S. (2013). Practical reason within and across disciplinary borders: A response to Longhofer and Floersch. *Research on Social Work Practice.* Advance online publication. doi:10.1177/1049731513509898

Kirk, S. A., & Reid, W. J. (2002). *Science and social work: A critical appraisal.* New York, NY: Columbia University Press.

Klein, J. T. (2004). Prospects for transdisciplinarity. *Futures, 36,* 515–526. doi:10.1016/j.futures.2003.10.007

Klein, J. T. (2008). Education. In G. Hirsch, H. Hoffmann-Riem, S. Biber-Klemm, W. Gossenbacher-Mansuy, D. Joye, C. Pohl, . . . E. Zemp (Eds.), *Handbook of transdisciplinary research* (pp. 399–410). Dordrecht, the Netherlands: Springer.

Klein, J. T. (2014). Communication and collaboration in interdisciplinary research. In M. O'Rourke, S. Crowley, S. D. Eigenbrode, & J. D. Wulfhorst (Eds.), *Enhancing communication & collaboration in interdisciplinary research* (pp. 11–30). Thousand Oaks, CA: Sage.

Krettek, A., & Thorpenberg, S. (2011, January). Transdisciplinary higher education—A challenge for public health science. *Education Research International.* http://dx.doi.org/10.1155/2011/649539

Larson, E. L., Landers, T. F., & Begg, M. D. (2011). Building interdisciplinary research models: A didactic course to prepare interdisciplinary scholars and faculty. *Clinical & Translational Science, 4,* 38–41. doi:10.1111/j.1752-8062.2010.00258.x

Lyall, C., Bruce, A., Tait, J., & Meagher, L. (2011). *Interdisciplinary research journeys: Practical strategies for capturing creativity.* New York: Bloomsbury Academic.

Lyall, C., & Meagher, L. R. (2012). A masterclass in interdisciplinarity: Research into practice in training the next generation of interdisciplinary researchers. *Futures, 44,* 608–617. doi:10.1016/j.futures.2012.03.011

Lyall, C., Meagher, L., & Tait, J. (2008). *A short guide to supervising interdisciplinary PhDs. ISSTI Briefing Note* (Number 4). Retrieved from http://www.issti.ed.ac.uk/__data/assets/file/0008/77606/ISSTI_Briefing_note_4_ID_supervision.pdf

Manathunga, C., Lant, P., & Mellick, G. (2006). Imagining an interdisciplinary doctoral pedagogy. *Teaching in Higher Education, 11,* 365–379. doi:10.1080/13562510600680954

Mech, M. H. (2001). Intellectual border crossing in graduate education: A report from the field. *Educational Researcher, 30*(5), 12–18.

Millar, M. M. (2013). Interdisciplinary research and the early career: The effect of interdisciplinary dissertation research on career placement and publication productivity of doctoral graduates in the sciences. *Research Policy, 42,* 1152–1164. doi:10.1016/j.respol.2013.02.004

Misra, S., Stokols, D., Hall, K., & Feng, A. (2011). Transdisciplinary training in health research: Distinctive features and future directions. In M. Kirst, N. Schaefer-McDaniel, S. Hwang, & P. O'Campo (Eds.), *Converging disciplines: A transdisciplinary research approach to urban health problems* (pp. 133–147). New York, NY: Springer.

Mitchell, C. A. (Ed.). (2009). *Quality in interdisciplinary and transdisciplinary postgraduate research and its supervision: Ideas for good practice.* Paper prepared for LTC Fellowship: Zen and the art of transdisciplinary postgraduate studies. Sydney, Australia: Institute for Sustainable Futures, University of Technology.

Mitrany, M., & Stokols, D. (2005). Gauging the transdisciplinary qualities and outcomes of doctoral training programs. *Journal of Planning Education and Research, 24,* 437–449. doi:10.1177/0739456X04270368

Mor Barak, M., & Brekke, J. S. (2014). Social work science and identity formation for doctoral scholars within intellectual communities. *Research on Social Work Practice.* Advance online publication. doi:10.1177/1049731514528047

Nash, J. M. (2008). Transdisciplinary training: Key components and prerequisites for success. *American Journal of Preventive Medicine, 35,* S133–S140. doi:10.1016/j.amepre.2008.05.004

Neuhauser, L., Richardson, D., Mackenzie, S., & Minkler, M. (2007). Advancing transdisciplinary and translational research practice: Issues and models of doctoral education in public health. *Journal of Research Practice, 3*(2), 1–24.

Nurius, P. S., & Kemp, S. P. (2013). Transdisciplinarity and translation: Preparing social work doctoral students for high impact research. *Research on Social Work Practice.* Advance online publication. doi:10.1177/1049731513512375

Nurius, P. S., & Kemp, S. P. (2014). Transdisciplinary and translational research. In C. Franklin (Ed.), *Encyclopedia of social work online*. NASW & Oxford University Press. doi:10.1093/acrefore/9780199975839.013.1060

Oliver, C. (2013). Social workers as boundary spanners: Reframing our professional identity for interprofessional practice. *Social Work Education: The International Journal, 32*, 773–784. doi:10.1080/02615479.2013.765401

Olivero, O. A. (2014). *Interdisciplinary mentoring in science: Strategies for success.* New York, NY: Academic Press.

Pallas, A. M. (2001). Preparing education doctoral students for epistemological diversity. *Educational Researcher, 30*(5), 1–6. doi:10.3102/0013189X030005006

Rosenfield, P. L. (1992). The potential of transdisciplinary research for sustaining and extending linkages between the health and social sciences. *Social Science & Medicine, 35*, 1343–1357. doi:10.1016/0277-9536(92)90038-R

Schmidt, A. H., Robbins, A. S. T., Combs, J. K., Freeburg, A., Jesperson, R. G., Rogers, H. S., . . . Wheat, E. (2012). A new model for training graduate students to conduct interdisciplinary, interorganizational and international research. *BioScience, 62*, 296–304. doi:10.1525/bio.2012.62.3.11

Schnapp, L. M., Rotschy, L., Hall, T. E., Crowley, S., O'Rourke, & O'Rourke, M. (2012). How to talk to strangers: Facilitating knowledge sharing within translational health teams with the Toolbox dialogue method. *Translational Behavioral Medicine, 2*, 469–479. doi:10.1007/s13142-012-0171-2

Society for Social Work and Research Strategic Plan 2012–2017. Retrieved from http://www.sswr.org/SSWR%20Strategic%20Plan-2012-2017.pdf.

Stokols, D. (2006). Toward a science of transdisciplinary action research. *American Journal of Community Psychology, 38*, 63–77. doi:10.1007/s10464-006-9060-5

Stokols, D. (2014). Training the next generation of transdisciplinarians. In M. O'Rourke, S. Crowley, S. D. Eigenbrode, & J. D. Wulfhorst (Eds.), *Enhancing communication & collaboration in interdisciplinary research* (pp. 56–81). Los Angeles, CA: Sage.

Tötzer, T., Sedlacek, S., & Knoflacher, M. (2011). Designing the future: A reflection of a transdisciplinary case study in Austria. *Futures, 43*, 840–852. doi:10.1016/j.futures.2011.05.026

Wagner, T., Baum, L., & Newbill, P. (2013). From rhetoric to real world: Fostering higher order thinking through transdisciplinary collaboration. *Innovations in Education and Teaching International.* Advance online publication. doi:10.1080/14703297.2013.796726

Willetts, J., & Mitchell, C. (2006, 3–6 December). *Learning to be a "transdisciplinary" sustainability researcher: A community of practice approach.* Proceedings of the 12th ANZSYS Conference—Sustaining our social and natural capital, Katoomba, NSW, Australia.

# Applying Sociocultural Theory to Teaching Statistics for Doctoral Social Work Students

CRISTINA MOGRO-WILSON, MICHAEL G. REEVES,
and MOLLIE LAZAR CHARTER

*School of Social Work, University of Connecticut, West Hartford, Connecticut, USA*

*This article describes the development of two doctoral-level multivariate statistics courses utilizing sociocultural theory, an integrative pedagogical framework. In the first course, the implementation of sociocultural theory helps to support the students through a rigorous introduction to statistics. The second course involves students developing and testing their own hypotheses on secondary data sets, writing conference abstracts, and presenting at a mock conference. Quantitative and qualitative data from student feedback highlight the impact of this course, and findings from a short survey of doctoral programs suggest the widespread need for an effective approach to teaching doctoral-level statistics. The course model presented can be easily implemented in other doctoral programs of social work.*

## INTRODUCTION

The capability of doctoral programs to produce highly proficient researchers is essential for the continuation and growth of our profession. In addition to becoming educators for BSW and MSW students, graduates of doctoral programs contribute to building the social work literature and knowledge base that is utilized in helping vulnerable and marginalized populations. Nationally, there is widespread concern about the effectiveness of social work doctoral programs at preparing their graduates for jobs in academia (Dinerman, Feldman, & Ello, 1999; Karger & Stoesz, 2003; Valentine et al.,

151

1998). Although most doctoral programs in social work have preparation for academic employment as one of the goals, and the majority of doctoral students state that they will be seeking academic jobs (Dinerman et al., 1999), the amount of curricular attention devoted to developing skills necessary for a fruitful academic career is limited.

Students may not feel that they are receiving adequate statistical knowledge in their doctoral programs. In a study of more than 800 doctoral students, the most commonly cited curricular concern was about research, with some students citing specific concerns about the lack of applicability of their statistics classes to their work. Other concerns included a discontentment with having to take statistics courses *outside* of the school of social work (Anastas, 2012).

There are also general concerns in social work about how well some doctoral programs prepare their graduates for scholarly productivity (Karger & Stoesz, 2003). For example, in a study that included the majority of all social work doctoral graduates from American universities during a 28-year period, one third of graduates had not made any presentations at professional social work conferences (Abbott, 1985). Doctoral programs should provide students with opportunities to apply for funding, write abstracts, present at conferences, and write manuscripts for publication—all experiences that may increase their productivity after graduation.

Currently, there are no specific curricular requirements for social work doctoral programs. The Group for the Advancement of Doctoral Education has created guidelines outlining a vision for social work education that includes research training (http://www.gadephd.org/). However, the Group for the Advancement of Doctoral Education guidelines do not identify the specific curricular elements that will likely lead doctoral students to become skilled researchers. Further, the 1991 findings of the National Institute of Mental Health's Task Force on Social Work Research found that much of the research reported in social work journals had low internal validity and neglected the use of adequate statistical techniques, illustrating the critical need for comprehensive statistical training. Other social work scholars have called for educational reform to better equip social work researchers with current methodological tools (Fraser, Jenson, & Lewis, 1993; Howard, Himle, Jenson, & Vaughn, 2009; Khinduka, 2002).

A 2006 annual survey of 69 social work doctoral programs in the United States indicated that there is a growing need for literature on teaching statistics to doctoral students (Council on Social Work Education Commission on Accreditation, 2006). An extensive literature search on teaching doctoral statistics in social work provided no articles on this topic; however, there are many articles on teaching statistics to social work students in master's degree programs (Forte, 1995; Lazar, 1990; McCoyd, Johnson, Munch, & LaSala, 2009; Wells, 2006). Educators in the field of statistics recognize that it is difficult for all students to learn statistical and mathematical procedures (Watts, 1991) and that change is necessary in how it is taught (Hogg, 1991; Ojeda & Sosa, 2002; Snee, 1993). The pedagogy of statistics in the social sciences remains underdeveloped and is often taught in a monologic or banking approach (Helmericks, 1993) via lecture, homework assignments, and test taking.

In this article, we suggest that requiring two doctoral courses in introductory and advanced multivariate statistics, which utilize applied methods and a sociocultural framework, represents a concrete step toward assuring that the profession will have well-trained researchers and academics. The goal of this article is to introduce a theoretical framework and pedagogical tool that has been used in two courses, Multivariate Statistics I and II. The primary objectives of the course are to teach basic and advanced statistics while allowing doctoral students to develop and test their own hypotheses on secondary data sets. Moreover, the main focus of the second course is for the student to produce and submit a conference abstract to the Society for Social Work Research (SSWR), as well as give it as an oral presentation to the class. The courses were implemented at the University of Connecticut School of Social Work in the 2011–2012 academic year, using an innovative teaching framework focused on application, integration with statistical software, and development of skills. This article includes the development of the course, its areas of emphasis, and the multiple modes of delivery. The authors believe that the techniques described are easily adapted for in other doctoral social work programs.

## THEORETICAL FRAMEWORK

Sociocultural theory provides an integrative pedagogical framework that was utilized in the development of these courses (Vygotsky, 1978). The sociocultural framework is a constructivist theory of learning, which suggests that all higher learning occurs in the framework of significant relationships and that learning best occurs when students work alongside a more knowledgeable individual such as a teacher, mentor, or more experienced peer, who will be able to offer direction. Vygotsky (1978) outlined the zone of proximal development (ZPD), which is "the distance between the actual developmental level as determined by independent problem solving and the level of potential development as determined through problem solving under adult guidance or in collaboration with more capable peers" (p. 89). In other words, Vygotsky indicated that it would be incomplete to only examine students' current and independent capability, but rather one must look to their potential learning capability within a social context. Aptly, he suggested, "the actual developmental level characterizes mental development *retrospectively*, while the zone of proximal development characterizes mental development *prospectively* [emphasis added] (Vygotsky, 1978, p. 89). The ZPD indicates the potential that students have to learn within a social context.

Central to sociocultural theory is the suggestion that learning takes place within a social context, that a social context is "the total life space in which individual development takes place" and can include a variety of elements, such as family, community, and factors related to diversity such as race and gender (Alfred, 2002, p. 7). Learning occurs in many areas of life, and "through acting on things in the world [people] engage with the meanings that those things assumed within social activity" (Daniels, 2001, p. 56). In other words, students exist within a cultural context and, therefore, that learning occurs socially, as well as within a classroom. The implications for the present study are an awareness of diverse social contexts within which students exist and the importance of learning as a social activity, both with an instructor and colleagues. Therefore, the most important work done by an educator is to create a ZPD through implementing effective scaffolding, or the use of flexible structures and supports offered by a mentor or teacher to facilitate learning (Hasse, 2001).

## Theoretical Application

According to Daniels (2001), Vygotsky's ZPD framework suggests at least two important pedagogical elements: First, students should be assessed by their potential for learning rather than their actual and demonstrated knowledge, and second, a central task of education is to "create the possibilities for development, through the kind of active participation that characterizes collaboration, that it should be socially negotiated, and that it should entail transfer of control to the learner" (p. 61). The course enrollment was both 1st- and 2nd-year students with varying degrees of computer, mathematical, and statistical experience. However, the students' knowledge was less important than their potential for learning.

The first task of the first course is to develop an atmosphere of support, in which scaffolding can be erected to encourage students to learn within their ZPD. Flexible structures work to create a comfortable learning environment with a pedagogical focus on making the material accessible to all students and on developing a mutual respect between the instructor and students. Additional methods that worked to increase comfort for students included presenting material to the students with humor, sharing vignettes about academic experiences, and encouraging questions about the course and academic life. Flexible supports were implemented, and students were given the opportunity to complete homework independently and then review it in class without grading repercussions so that they would be able to improve their confidence with statistical analyses, and explore their learning potential, without being concerned about their grades.

Another important element of the course was to continually underscore the practical application of statistics and the usefulness of the course material for the students' future careers. By focusing on students' future careers and by allowing them to select their own research foci in the second semester, students took an active collaborative role with the instructor, because power over learning, in fact, largely rested with them. Focused attention was given to the application of each statistical method in academic research, thereby ensuring that students understood not only the material presented but also how it might be used during their careers. The applicability of course material was reinforced through requiring that students find articles in the literature that implemented the statistical methods covered in class and by requiring each one to create a binder containing all materials from the course, organized by statistical method, with the stated purpose being a reference for future research endeavors. By focusing on the practical application of statistics in their future careers, positive regard was increased, self-confidence enhanced, and usefulness of statistics made explicit.

Use of interactive lectures and cooperative learning strategies also has been shown to enhance the learning process. Interactive lectures are a time-honored technique that allows teachers to engage students and enhance learning in the classroom (Consortium for the Advancement of Undergraduate Statistics Education [CAUSE], https://www.causeweb.org/). In our model, the instructor used direct classroom demonstration of SPSS, practice in the campus computer lab, and students' presentations of their own data analysis to enhance learning. In addition, cooperative learning strategies (such as structured small-group projects) made each students success dependent on the group's success. Students were given time to work as a group in class as well as expected to work together outside of class to complete their projects. These groups emphasized the five key elements of cooperative learning (https://www.causeweb.org/): positive interdependence, individual accountability, promotion of interaction, interpersonal and small-group social skills, and group processing.

In tandem with the flexible supports provided, the curriculum for the first semester—which consisted of a thorough review of research methodology, univariate and bivariate statistical methods and hands-on use of the principal statistical software—encouraged learning and helped each student to develop a working knowledge and command of the core methods. Under the guidance of the instructor, students with greater confidence and experience in theoretical and practical applications were able to mentor peers with less experience. By the end of the first semester, all students had developed the fundamental skills and confidence necessary to move to more complex tasks in the second semester, including the application of multivariate techniques to secondary data.

Hence, students entered the second semester with essential core knowledge and with a strong understanding of the symbols used in academic research. During this second semester, they were expected to apply this knowledge to their own research interests, conducting analyses on publicly available data sets. This teaching approach resulted in a significant expression of interest among the social work faculty, two of whom asked to take part in the courses. Their additional thoughts and support helped provide the scaffolding important in the application of sociocultural theory.

In addition to emphasizing the practical applicability of statistics, by encouraging students to apply analyses to their areas of interest, the instructor purposively used class time to engage students in discussion about the importance of statistical methods both in conducting research and in the process of entering academia. The instructor, a social work faculty member, emphasized how each statistical method could be applied to social work research specifically. In addition, as a recent graduate from a social work doctoral program, she had current knowledge of the job market, of the heavy demands of doctoral work, and of the need to ease students into academic culture. The instructor often used class time to develop rapport and relationships with the doctoral students in order to gain respect and positive regard and to help develop the mentor–student bond—central tenets of sociocultural theory.

Equally important, the instructor worked to develop the students' enjoyment of statistics. This was easier than anticipated: The instructor's passion for (and enjoyment of) statistics was easily communicated to the students, which made the information more compelling. In addition, students became more deeply engaged once they were able to apply statistical methods to their own research.

## DIDACTIC DESCRIPTION OF THE COURSES

The primary goal of the first-semester course was to introduce students to essential statistical analyses with a focus on learning how to conduct each analysis with SPSS software. Attention was placed on the purpose of each method and potential future uses of each analysis in academic research. Students in this course learned how to manipulate SPSS 22.0, using both a "point-and-click" technique and through syntax. With computer assistance, students learned to produce codebooks; generate frequency tables and graphs; and perform statistical analyses such as $t$ tests, chi-squares, correlations, analyses of variance, and multiple regressions.

Classroom lectures were presented in PowerPoint, utilizing humor and comical graphics as much as possible; class discussions reviewed the theoretical aspects of the techniques, whereas demonstrations focused on the practical elements of each, such as the interpretation and use of results. The typical format of the PowerPoint presentations was to describe the statistical method and the underlying theory, as well as to convey the uses of the statistical test and what assumptions need to be met to perform a particular analysis. Next, the point-and-click technique in SPSS was covered, as well as how to read and conduct the analysis in the syntax. Finally, how to interpret the output from SPSS and write up the findings was reviewed. Students were given handouts of the PowerPoint presentations, the syntax, and the output with step-by-step annotations regarding how to interpret the findings. These handouts also were posted on the class Blackboard site. In addition, students were given homework in which they were expected to practice the analyses covered in class.

During the first course, students continued learning statistical techniques through creating and testing the reliability of scales and learning how to deal with missing data. As noted, correlation, $t$ tests, and chi-square were practiced using example data. Once students were comfortable with these bivariate techniques, analysis of variance and analyses of covariance were introduced. They then were asked to pick interesting variables from practice data sets to analyze.

The primary textbook used was Abu-Bader (2011). The SPSS survival manual by Pallant (2010) also proved to be an extremely accessible text for direct application of the concepts for SPSS users. In addition, Tabachnick and Fidell's (2007) book was introduced as a resource and was used as the primary text in the second semester, and Allison's (1999) primer on multiple regression provided helpful course examples. The first semester concluded with multiple regression. (See Table 1 for the content of the first semester.)

Assignments during this first course emphasized data analyses in order to provide experience in working with the SPSS program. Practice using the program is essential but should not override the more important focus on theory and hypothesis construction. We decided that class discussions should be oriented primarily to conceptual and theoretical concerns, whereas the assignments would be mostly technical. Through assignments that required students to perform technical analyses, and to write up their findings, they practiced the techniques they eventually will be using as teachers, researchers, and scholars. In addition, they were asked to find an article (or part of a dissertation) in their area of interest that presented a similar analysis. These homework assignments and articles became part of the binders that students developed, along with PowerPoint slides, notes, annotated syntax, and output provided by the instructor. Students also often volunteered to demonstrate and discuss their homework for the entire class.

We recognized that many doctoral students were expected to transition from the role of practitioner to the role of researcher (Mendenhall, 2007), and most had not had any statistical training since their MSW or BSW course of study. We acknowledged Dewey's (1947) method of teaching, which always includes students' experiences, where each student's learning needs are integrated with the curriculum. Life experiences, curiosity, and passion for an issue often are the driving factors that bring students into doctoral education; these courses utilized those very factors to motivate them to learn multivariate statistics. For these reasons, the second course was centered primarily on the interests of the students.

**TABLE 1** First Semester Statistics Course

| | |
|---|---|
| Week 1 | Introduction to the course; overview of research methods, the nature of causality, levels of measurement |
| | Creating a codebook |
| Week 2 | Distributions and descriptives; central tendency and dispersion (variance and standard deviation); Kurtosis and Skewness |
| | Creating an SPSS data file, entering data, and cleaning data |
| Week 3 | Sampling distributions—sample size and error; standard scores |
| | Graphs in SPSS and moving them to word documents |
| Week 4 | Manipulation of the data: reverse scoring items, collapsing continuous and categorical variables |
| | Creating scales; checking reliability of a scale |
| | Finding and dealing with outliers |
| | Dealing with non-normality; transforming skewed variables, bootstrapping |
| Week 5 | Correlation |
| | Partial correlation |
| | Selecting the right statistical test |
| Week 6 | t tests (one sample t test, independent samples t test, & paired samples t test) |
| | Chi-square goodness of fit & chi-square test for independence |
| Week 7 | One way between-groups ANOVA |
| | One-way between-groups ANOVA with planned comparisons |
| | Repeated-measures ANOVA (within-subjects) |
| Week 8 | Two-way between-groups ANOVA |
| | Mixed between-within ANOVA |
| | Interaction effects (spuriousness, confounding, suppression, mediation, moderation . . .) |
| Weeks 9, 10, 11 | Multiple regression |
| | Major assumptions of multiple regression |
| Week 12 | Dummy coding |
| | Hierarchical multiple regression |
| | Interpreting regression in the literature |
| Week 13 | Missing data |
| | Sample weight |
| | Interpreting regression tables |
| Week 14 | Review of regression |
| | Finding a secondary data set |

ANOVA = analysis of variance.

In Multivariate Statistics II, students were encouraged to explore data repositories, such as the Interuniversity Consortium for Political and Social Research (n.d.) at the University of Michigan (http://www.icpsr.umich.edu/icpsrweb/ICPSR/access/index.jsp) during the semester break in order to find a data set of interest to them to work with during the second semester. In addition, students were given other websites that house datasets such as Sociometrics (http://www.socio.com/data.php), the U.S. Department of Education (http://nces.ed.gov/das/), the U.S. Department of Health and Human Services Centers for Disease Control and Prevention (http://www.cdc.gov/datastatistics/), and the U.S. National Institutes of Health National Library of Medicine (http://www.nlm.nih.gov/hsrinfo/datasites.html).

Students presented the data sets they found and were given the option of working individually or in small groups. Several students chose to work in pairs or groups, supporting the main tenet of sociocultural theory, which is that all higher learning occurs in the framework of significant relationships. Individuals and teams identified specific research questions they hoped to address with the data. One group of students chose to work with the Center for Disease Control's 2007 National Health Interview Survey, to investigate the impact of different variables on utilization of complementary and alternative medicine practices. They found that higher educational levels and better insurance were positively correlated with higher complementary and alternative medicine usage. An individual student utilized the National Criminal Justice Treatment Practices Survey of co-occurring substance use and mental disorder treatment services in criminal justice settings (2002–2008) to investigate transition planning and community collaboration. A student group chose to use the 2007 Baylor Religion Survey data to look at the relationship between multicultural exposure, religiosity, and acceptance of interracial marriage. An additional student utilized the Cingranelli-Richards Human Rights Dataset, World Bank Development Indicators, CIA World Fact Book, and the Armed Conflict Dataset to test a model for urban water access. Furthermore, one student decided to collect her own data on the perception of feminism among MSW candidates (Charter, 2015).

Students conducted literature reviews and discussed their interests, research questions, and hypotheses in class, and then began the task of cleaning their data, as they had learned during the first semester. Concurrently, they continued to practice more complex statistical analyses, including ANCOVA, MANCOVA, logistic regression, and factor analysis, and then were introduced to structural equation modeling and hierarchical linear modeling (see Table 2). Special attention was given to analyses that students hoped to use when working with their data sets. Students finished the semester by conducting analyses of their data and writing an abstract to be submitted to the SSWR and presented to their classmates.

Of the 10 social work students enrolled in the second-semester course, all but one submitted an abstract to the SSWR 2012 conference. Two of the abstracts submitted were accepted, and presented at the SSWR 2012 conference. In addition, three of the students submitted their (slightly modified) abstracts to other conferences, and all three were accepted. Further, one student has a manuscript in press based on the research and findings she conducted during the course (Charter, 2015). This student had surveyed an MSW student population about their perceptions of feminists and completed appropriate statistical analyses, which indicated important findings related to student feminist self-identification. Moreover, at least two more students were planning to submit their findings to peer-reviewed journals. In addition to these achievements, perhaps the greatest accomplishment was the students' enjoyment of statistics, about which many of them spoke freely.

**TABLE 2** Second Semester Statistics Course

| | |
|---|---|
| Week 1 | Introduction to the course |
| | Overviews of Multivariate Stats I |
| | Establishing a substantive interest |
| Week 2 | Concept mapping |
| | Getting a secondary data set in shape for analysis |
| Week 3 | Remembering multiple regression |
| | Operationalizing your concept map |
| Weeks 4 & 5 | One-way analysis of covariance |
| | Two-way analysis of covariance |
| Week 6 | Multivariate analysis of variance |
| | Multivariate analysis of covariance |
| Weeks 7 & 8 | Logistic regression |
| Week 9 | Principal components analysis |
| | Factor analysis |
| Week 10 | Hierarchical linear modeling |
| Week 11 | Structural equation modeling |
| Week 12 | Go over homework assignments |
| | Overview of census data and social explorer |
| | Writing for publication |
| | Interviewing for faculty positions |
| Weeks 13 & 14 | Student oral presentations "Mock SSWR" |

By using data that interested them, and that they selected, students were able to see the power of statistical analysis and how statistics could impact their own thinking and scholarship. By the end of the second semester, students who had started the academic year with greatly varying levels of under-standing and confidence in statistics all had produced submission-worthy abstracts, illustrating that the course had drawn upon their ZPDs, in which learning potential was maximized through collaborative work both with their instructor and peers.

## THE PRESENT STUDY METHOD

In response to the positive student feedback about these courses, and sub-sequently to finding a lack of literature about how to teach doctoral-level statistics in social work, the authors present the following course evaluations. The quantitative and qualitative course evaluations from the two statistics courses were analyzed to better glean a picture of student experiences in the course. Student evaluations of the courses were conducted using quantitative and qualitative survey methods at the end of each semester.

## RESULTS

Standard university-wide course evaluations (utilizing quantitative and qual-itative questions) were conducted at the end of the semester and were used to evaluate the course. The quantitative element consisted of 10 questions self-administered by the student on a Likert-style scale of 1 to 10, ranging from *unacceptable* to *outstanding*. The questions asked about presentation of material; organization of class; clear objectives; fulfilled objectives; clear assignments; stimulated interest; fair grading; and the accessibility, preparation, and interest of the instructor. The fall 2011 course with 10 students had an overall rating of 9.7 out of 10. This may be compared to the mean ratings of the department of 9.3 and the mean rating for the university of 9.2. The spring 2012 course with 11 students (there was one student from another discipline) had an overall rating of 9.7. This can be compared to the mean ratings of the department of 9.3 and the mean rating for the university of 9.3.

The open-ended qualitative questions inquired about the most useful aspect of the course, what could be improved, and if there were specific suggestions for improvement. Qualitative data were analyzed for 10 students (combining responses from fall 2011 and spring 2012).

Four major themes emerged. First, the personality of the instructor was reported to be very important to the learning process. Most students felt that the professor's ability to bring her persona to the classroom presentations made her approachable and the material less intimidating. Students felt the positive, engaging style of interaction of the instructor, and her enthusiasm for the material, helped make the topic approachable. Second, the clear expectations presented for each class helped students to feel prepared. Third, the use of PowerPoint presentations, explicit demonstrations with SPSS, and follow-up on homework assignments all were reported as positive pedagogies of the course. Students felt that continuing the development of a binder from each week's assignment would be beneficial in the future. Fourth, students felt that the assignments were not just academic exercises but would be helpful for their future dissertations and publishing.

Students also suggested areas for improvement. The major theme that emerged was to slow down and take more time for questions to ensure that students with differing academic backgrounds could keep up with the material. Some suggested the integration of more published research into the discussions and more in-class homework review. On a more practical level, students suggested that the class be held in a computer lab that would provide access to SPSS for each student.

## CHALLENGES

Few major challenges arose during the implementation of this course, but one minor challenge was that, although the instructor presented the possible future application of the statistical methods throughout the first semester, it was not until students began to utilize their found data sets that they seemed to fully comprehend how the statistical analyses could be used with the data. The students presented as being excited about work with their data sets during the second semester because they were given the opportunity to choose data sets that were of interest to them. Through trial and error they learned which statistical methods would best accommodate their variables and research questions. Utilizing actual (rather than educational) data made the analyses somewhat more complicated, allowing for the generation of many and varied questions, which actually may more accurately reflect their future research. The implementation of this course, however, clearly will require instructors to be flexible and available to field student questions and concerns as they arise both in and out of the classroom.

Some students elected to create or collect their own data. Two students created their own data sets by combining several different sources, and one student chose to collect her own data. These processes were quite complex and required time during the winter break (prior to starting the second semester) to make sure the students were ready to fully engage in the second course. In addition, some of the data sets were gathered using complex sampling designs, in which the use of sampling weights became an issue. The students asked the doctoral committee to purchase an SPSS complex samples add-on package to deal with these issues, and the doctoral program provided the scaffolding and support to pay for this additional software.

## DISCUSSION

Developing a statistics course for doctoral social work students is a challenge, particularly because these students typically come with diverse epistemological backgrounds. Given that the literature offers limited solutions to this challenge, it is an area that requires much more exploration, research, and discussion. The authors hope that this article on incorporating sociocultural theory, interactive lectures, cooperative learning, and applied secondary data analysis into teaching statistics will be a catalyst for innovative change.

Utilizing sociocultural theory for the framework of teaching doctoral statistics proved useful for facilitating students' learning of statistics. It provided a degree of continuity throughout the semester while allowing students to test their own hypotheses. Interactive lectures keep them engaged, and the cooperative learning paradigm enhanced learning. The use of live secondary data sets (that had not been cleaned or perfected for in-class use) allowed the students to begin to recognize and struggle with issues regarding the reliability and validity of data. As a corollary, they also found themselves considering how their own assumptions might sometimes bias their research. Meanwhile, students took ownership of their ideas because they were testing their own hypotheses. The primary disadvantage was the time involved in constructing the database, although this limitation appears to be outweighed by the numerous overall advantages of the teaching method.

## FUTURE CONSIDERATIONS

Further data collection and analysis may enhance the generalizability of these preliminary findings. Satisfaction ratings from additional student cohorts would be important to review. A sophisticated tool, such as the Survey of Attitudes towards Statistics scale, could be used to further analyze the data collected on student attitudes gathered here using only a simple, universal school-wide tool (VanHoof, Kuppens, Castro Sotos, Verschaffel, & Onghena, 2011). Data on students' self-identified comfort level with statistics, computers, and mathematics prior to enrolling in (and after completing) the course would allow for further examination of the effectiveness of the model. Analysis also could be conducted on the impact of the model by comparing satisfaction ratings from years when a more monologic method was used at the same school, and among schools that use different models, and the satisfaction ratings when the course is taught by a social worker versus a statistician. Finally, game-based instructional techniques can be deployed to enhance classroom learning for typically dry subject areas (https://www.causeweb.org/). These and other techniques could be incorporated into the first semester to further increase the enjoyment of the classroom experience when the pedagogical focus of the model is on improving the students' self-confidence and enhancing their level of comfort.

## ACKNOWLEDGMENTS

We gratefully acknowledge Dr. Alex Gitterman, Director of the doctoral program, for supporting this innovative teaching methodology.

## REFERENCES

Abbott, A. (1985). Research productivity patterns of social work doctorates. *Social Work Research and Abstracts, 21*, 11–17. doi:10.1093/swra/21.3.11

Abu-Bader, S. H. (2011). *Using statistical methods in social science research with a complete SPSS guide*. Chicago, IL: Lyceum Books.

Alfred, M. V. (2002). The promise of sociocultural theory in democratizing adult education. In M. V. Alfred (Ed.), *Learning and sociocultural context: Implications for adults, community and workplace education* (pp. 3–13). San Francisco: Jossey Bass.

Allison, P. (1999). *Multiple regression: A primer*. Thousand Oaks, CA: Pine Forge.

Anastas, J. W. (2012). *Doctoral education in social work*. New York, NY: Oxford University Press.

Charter, M. L. (2015). Feminist self-identification among social work students. *Journal of Social Work Education, 51*, 72–89.

Council on Social Work Education Commission on Accreditation. (2006). *Statistics on social work education in the United States.* Alexandria, VA: Council on Social Work Education.

Daniels, H. (2001). *Vygotsky and pedagogy.* London, UK: Routledge/Falmer.

Dewey, J. (1947). *Experience and education.* New York, NY. Macmillan.

Dinerman, M., Feldman, P., & Ello, L. (1999). Preparing practitioners for the professoriate. *Journal of Teaching in Social Work, 18,* 23–32. doi:10.1300/J067v18n01_05

Forte, J. A. (1995). Teaching statistics without sadistics. *Journal of Social Work Education, 31,* 204–218.

Fraser, M. W., Jenson, J. M., & Lewis, R. E. (1993). Research training in social work: The continuum is not a continuum. *Journal of Social Work Education, 29,* 46–62.

Hasse, C. (2001). Institutional creativity: The relational zone of proximal development. *Culture & Psychology, 7,* 199–221. doi:10.1177/1354067X0172005

Helmericks, S. G. (1993). Collaborative testing in social statistics: Toward gemeinstat. *Teaching Sociology, 21,* 287–297. doi:10.2307/1319027

Hogg, R. V. (1991). Statistical education: Improvements are badly needed. *The American Statistician, 45,* 342–343.

Howard, M. Q., Himle, J., Jenson, J. M., & Vaughn, M. G. (2009). Revisioning social work clinical education: Recent developments in relation to evidence-based practice. *Journal of Evidence-Based Practice, 6,* 256–273.

Karger, H. J., & Stoesz, D. (2003). The growth of social work education programs, 1985-1999: Its impact on economic and educational factors related to the profession of social work. *Journal of Social Work Education, 39,* 279–285.

Khinduka, S. (2002). Musings on doctoral education in social work. *Research on Social Work Practice, 12,* 684–694. doi:10.1177/1049731502012005007

Lazar, A. (1990). Statistics course in social work education. *Journal of Teaching in Social Work, 4,* 17–30. doi:10.1300/J067v04n01_03

McCoyd, J. L. M., Johnson, Y. M., Munch, S., & LaSala, M. (2009). Quantocentric culture: Ramifications for social work education. *Social Work Education, 28,* 811–827. doi:10.1080/02615470802478238

Mendenhall, A. N. (2007). Switching hats: Transitioning from the role of clinician to the role of researcher in doctoral social work education. *Journal of Teaching in Social Work, 27,* 273–290. doi:10.1300/J067v27n03_17

Ojeda, M. M., & Sosa, V. (2002). An applied statistics course for systematics and ecology PhD students. *International Journal of Mathematical Education in Science and Technology, 33,* 199–211. doi:10.1080/00207390110113543

Pallant, J. (2010). *SPSS survival manual* (4th ed.). Crows Nest, Australia: Allen & Unwin.

Snee, R. D. (1993). What's missing in statistical education? *The American Statistician, 47,* 149–154.

Tabachnick, B. G., & Fidell, L. S. (2007). *Using multivariate statistics* (5th ed.). Boston, MA: Allyn & Bacon.

Valentine, D. P., Edwards, S., Gohagan, D., Huff, M., Pereira, A., & Wilson, P. (1998). Preparing social work doctoral students for teaching: Report of a survey. *Journal of Social Work Education, 34,* 273–282.

VanHoof, S., Kuppens, S., Castro Sotos, A. E., Verschaffel, L., & Onghena, P. (2011). Measuring statistics attitudes: Structure of the survey of attitudes towards statistics. *Statistic Education Research Journal*, *10*, 35–51.

Vygotsky, L. S. (1978). *Mind and society: The development of higher mental processes*. Cambridge, MA: Harvard University Press.

Watts, D. G. (1991). Why is introductory statistics difficult to learn? And what can we do to make it easier? *The American Statistician*, *45*, 290–291.

Wells, M. (2006). Teaching notes: Making statistics "real" for social work students. *Journal of Social Work Education*, *42*, 397–404. doi:10.5175/JSWE.2006. 200400466

# Challenges and Strategies in Social Work and Social Welfare PhD Education: Helping Candidates Jump Through the Dissertation Hoops

RONI BERGER

*School of Social Work, Adelphi University, Garden City, New York, USA*

*A major task of social work doctoral programs is preparing the next generation of researchers and educators in the profession. To develop competence in generating new knowledge relevant to social work practice and disseminating it to future practitioners, doctoral candidates need to master a broad and complicated set of theoretical, empirical, and pedagogical knowledge and skills. Acquiring the relevant information and capabilities is a demanding process. Specifically, developing a research proposal and completing a successful dissertation is a complex, multifaceted task. In the process of accomplishing this task, students encounter intellectual, logistic, and emotional challenges. The main resource for helping them shoulder these challenges is the advisor. Informed by many years of the author's service as a dissertation advisor, this article reviews the challenges and offers effective strategies that the advisor can use to help the students address them.*

Social work and social welfare doctoral programs are the incubators for the next generation of educators and scholars in the profession (Liechty, Liao, & Schull, 2009; Stoesz, Karger, & Carrilio, 2010). One aspect of this task is helping these students develop the knowledge and skills necessary to function competently as part of the academic community (Spring, 2010).

Activities of members of this community involve two major components—the generation of new knowledge in one's discipline by conducting research, and the education of the next generation of members of the profession. To maintain these two foci, the German philosopher Wilhelm Freiherr von Humboldt (1767–1835) advocated for the unity of research and education as the ideal and the involvement of teachers in higher education institutions in research and teaching as interconnected (Kornbeck, 2007).

The pull between the two tasks is particularly evident in professional schools because of their mission to educate future practitioners. Because social work is a profession, a major challenge in doctoral education is to help candidates embrace a dual mission: While developing comfort with moving between theoretical conceptualization and empirical research, they must keep practice in mind. This is particularly challenging for doctoral programs that emphasize the preparation of graduates who can effectively train practitioners (as well as contribute to the knowledge base of the profession) rather than disproportionally focus on the volume of publications and grants. The latter may compromise graduates' ability to make empirical knowledge applicable and useful for practitioners (Berger, 2010) and lead to a shortage of faculty who are well equipped to help BSW and MSW students properly apply the principles of evidence-based practice, and leave programs challenged in their efforts to recruit faculty who combine research knowledge with the experience needed to train competent practitioners.

Doctoral programs in social work and social welfare vary in their self-positioning on the research-teaching practitioners continuum. Programs that emphasize the former focus on fostering graduates' research competence and equipping them with the ability to produce a large number of publications in prominent refereed journals and to secure grants for funded research; programs that underscore the latter concentrate on fostering graduates' pedagogical knowledge and teaching competence.

These differences in emphasis are manifested in the availability of and tension between PhD and DSW programs. In spite of these differences, all doctoral programs face the complex task of helping their students reach a higher level of learning and develop their ability to synthesize existing information, build on this synthesis to develop new ideas, and ultimately create and disseminate new knowledge relevant for the mission of the discipline (Spring, 2010).

Challenges involved in accomplishing this complex task can be conceptualized by applying Bloom's (1956) dynamic model of learning. His pyramid-shape six-tiered taxonomy of educational objectives includes increasing levels of thinking according to the degree of complexity required. At the base is knowledge of factual information, on which comprehension, application, analysis, synthesis, and evaluation are built hierarchically, such that a learner who functions on a "higher" level is assumed to have mastered "lower" levels. Although the taxonomy has been critiqued (Wineburg

& Schneider, 2010), it has been applied to fields as diverse as mathematics, English, chemistry, and nursing in a broad range of educational systems worldwide (Ferguson, 2002, Spring, 2010). A revised version presents the taxonomy as a two-dimensional model with a knowledge dimension referring to factual, conceptual, procedural, and metacognitive aspects and a cognitive process dimension referring to the activities required: remembering, understanding, applying, analyzing, evaluating, and creating (Anderson & Krathwohl, 2001; Krathwohl, 2002).

Related and somewhat similar to Bloom's taxonomy is the seven pillars paradigm of learning, which was developed in the early 1990 by the Society of College National and University Libraries (2007). The model is progressive and is designed to help gradually develop the learner's expertise in recognizing information needs; identifying and matching an information source with the specific information need; constructing search strategies that best reflect the information need; locating, accessing, and evaluating available information; organizing, applying, communicating, and synthesizing it; and building on it to create new knowledge (Spring, 2010).

The revised taxonomy and the Society of College National and University Libraries (SCONUL, 2007) model offer a useful lens to conceptualize the requirement of doctorate candidates to build on their master's-level competency in social work or related fields (e.g., public administration, public health, sociology, psychology) for critical and ethical application of available knowledge to client situations in the human services, in accordance with the principles of evidence-based practice (Council of Social Work Education [CSWE], 2008), and expand their expertise to include the ability to conduct and disseminate independent research in order to add to the knowledge base of the profession. By doing so, they can reach the highest level of creation, which includes the ability to put "elements together to form a coherent or functional whole; and reorganizing elements into a new pattern or structure through generating, planning, or producing" (Anderson & Krathwohl, 2001, pp. 67–68).

The demand to develop an ability to address higher levels of complexity as well as competency to disseminate this knowledge presents challenges to doctoral candidates and to the faculty who accompany them on their intellectual journey. Nowhere are these challenges more evident than in the development of a research proposal, the execution of the study, and the writing of the dissertation. At this final phase, candidates are expected to demonstrate more independence, and an ability to process knowledge and develop innovative ideas, than in any other part of the program, such as course work, comprehensive exams, qualifying paper, or other tasks used by programs to assess students understanding, proficiency, and readiness for this final step.

Previous authors have focused on student participation in writing groups to enhance the development of scholarly writing skills of students (Aitchison,

2009), the roles of the advisor (Spillett & Moisiewicz, 2004), and survival strategies reported by doctoral candidates (Mays & Smith, 2009). Focusing specifically on doctoral education in social work, Jenson (2008) emphasized the role of doctoral programs as the conduit for the development of skilled researchers and reviewed the challenges currently faced by programs. Anastas and Kuerbis (2009) studied the motivation, employment, and contributions of doctoral education to the profession and stated that "despite the fact that the first doctoral degree in social work was awarded in the 1920s, relatively little has been published about the characteristics of doctoral students and doctoral graduates in social work" (p. 72). Finally, Liechty et al. (2009) reviewed personal, relational, and structural factors affecting dissertation completion and offered strategies for facilitation, and Gordon (2003) provided advice for avoiding and coping with dissertation "hang-ups."

Based on this author's experience in teaching doctoral courses and overseeing dissertations, this article discusses challenges in helping doctoral candidates in social work and social welfare through the process of developing a proposal and completing a successful dissertation. Strategies for addressing these challenges are offered and illustrated.

## CHALLENGES

Along the journey toward developing a successful dissertation, intellectual, logistic, and emotional challenges present themselves and may contribute to doctoral program attrition. Data show that about half of students who begin a doctoral education fail to complete it (Liechty et al., 2009).

### Intellectual Challenges

In developing a credible research question and a research plan, students must think on a more sophisticated and independent level than before, and move comfortably between abstract ideas and their "translation" into a relevant and feasible theory-informed research agenda. Applying Bloom's taxonomy, they gradually must build on their factual knowledge and comprehension—which are required early in professional education—and application, which is the cornerstone of evidence-based practice, to demonstrate the ability to analyze, synthesize, and evaluate. Although these skills are also part of master's-level studies, they should be brought to fruition and be well developed at the doctoral level.

To this end, it is critical that students master the competence of "toying" intellectually with different conceptual frameworks and research approaches, "digest" relevant bodies of knowledge, and develop a picture of how different pieces of the process fit together. Furthermore, they also must learn to articulate a step-by-step argument in a scholarly style. Doctoral students need to gain intellectual flexibility when choosing a theory (or theories) that can best inform their research and the interpretation of their findings. We know that each research question can be approached from different theoretical angles and the choice of a particular approach affects the variables, constructs, and questions that are studied.

A related conceptual challenge is the need to "think big and act small." Students must combine a sound understanding of an issue from a theoretical perspective, sometimes integrating several conceptual frameworks to frame their question, with funneling the focus toward a practical plan for researching a very specific empirical question, which is feasible within the time and financial constraints of a doctoral program. In addition, they should be able to present a compelling argument for the significance of their research in light of its potential contribution to professional knowledge. To this end, they must be able to identify and position their own research question within the broader bodies of relevant knowledge from social work, social welfare, and related fields. Moreover, they need to understand diverse theories and their applicability to research, become familiar with positivistic and constructivist paradigms, and demonstrate comfort with diverse approaches to quantitative and qualitative research methods. These tasks often prove challenging for students and may require advisors to help them to identify the broad domains, which can inform their particular focus of interest. For example, a candidate interested in the relationships between the academic success of middle school students from minority groups and their perception of their teachers' attitudes toward them struggled with deciding which field to focus on. Should she review available knowledge about the nature and correlate of academic success in all age groups and with all topics? Should she delve into the ocean of developmental literature relative to characteristics of early adolescence, in general, or focus on the context of minority status, in particular? Which content, regarding the meaning of relationships in a cultural context, is required to effectively inform her study?

The move from the master's to PhD level requires a quantum leap in thinking about knowledge. Whereas the master's degree requires the development of an ability for critically evaluating and applying available knowledge to address the needs of client systems of all sizes, doctoral education is focused on the development of an ability to generate new knowledge valuable to practice and effectively disseminate such knowledge via publications, presentations, and teaching. Such different tasks require disparate ways of thinking and approaches, which are quite dissimilar. Rather than focusing on what is known, students are expected to learn to think about what is not known and to identify gaps in the available knowledge in order to address one of these gaps in their study. The challenge involved in this expectation was evident in a recent discussion with a student who was struggling to develop her research question. After canvassing the literature, she concluded that because nothing had been well studied relative to her specific topic of interest, she would need to abort it. It required quite an intensive mentoring process to help her and her classmates realize that this gap in knowledge was an excellent rationale for the significance of her question and that relevant literature to inform the conceptualization of her question should include studies on issues adjacent to her topic. In fact, the ready availability of studies of her specific question would nullify the need for an additional study of what was already explored.

The challenge for the educator in successfully accomplishing the transition to thinking like a doctoral student (while building on knowledge acquired in earlier professional education and practice) becomes finding an effective way to guide candidates in "expanding" their thinking to include both practice and research knowledge, and to develop their ability to "translate" theories of human development and human service intervention into a road map to inform their research.

## Logistic Challenges

There are several logistic challenges. The first is developing a realistic time (and financial) plan, based on an understanding of the process and the demands involved, and balancing the requirements of the program with other personal and professional responsibilities. To develop a realistic assessment of the amount of time and effort that each phase of the process requires, students must understand the diverse elements of the program, such as coursework, qualifying exams, or other gatekeeping program-specific requirements along the way, followed by the development of an approved proposal and the successful completion of a dissertation. They also must be well informed about all the steps involved in each element, their sequencing, time frames, and the decisions involved. For example, students typically are aware of the need to have approval from an Institutional Review Board before they start collecting data; however, some know only vaguely when they should seek the approval, how long it may take, and that this will require them to learn a tutorial and then be able to present documentation that they successfully passed an online exam. In addition, they will be expected to provide electronic and hard copies of the proposal in a format appropriate to the university's template, following a specified timetable. Similarly, students must be cognizant of available resources to support the cost of the program (e.g., stipends, research assistantships, adjunct teaching, types of registration [with or without advisement]), their financial and logistic implications, and conditions and procedures for requesting leaves of absence and medical leaves.

Because in social work and social welfare doctoral programs students typically are female, older, and involved in a professional career; have family responsibilities, and tend to be enrolled part time, a considerable balancing act may be required (Sussman, Stoddart, & Gorman, 2004). Moreover, students from historically underrepresented groups compose 40.1% of those taking coursework (CSWE, 2012). One third of those completing their doctoral education are age 45 or older (CSWE, 2012); many work in professional positions as practitioners or in administrative positions, have families, frequently have to care for children and elderly parents with health issues, and run a household. Consequently, they struggle to fit schoolwork, reading, research, and writing papers into an already tight schedule. In addition, because not all programs provide sufficient financial support, doctoral education often involves a fiscal strain, and opportunities that can help lighten the financial burden, such as adjunct teaching and research assistantships, further intensify the demands on candidates' time, often creating a vicious circle of stress.

## Emotional Challenges

The aforementioned challenges often create feelings of being overwhelmed. The multiple roles noted may also create contrasting role identities (Sussman et al., 2004), which may generate role conflict and role confusion. Although the whole process is stressful, some intersections are potentially more so. As the deadline for an approved proposal approaches, for example, and the possibility that all the sacrifice of effort, time, and money may lead to an ABD ("all but dissertation") status, frustration and sometimes anger and despair may settle in. Data from a study of pivotal points for dropping from doctoral programs across disciplines suggest that the dissertation phase is a high-risk period for attrition (Di Pierro, 2007).

The emotional toll involved in the development of a dissertation may beget anxiety, fear, self-doubt, loneliness, and disillusion. This presents to the advisor the challenge of offering support without compromising standards. A similar peak may occur during the writing of the discussion chapter of the dissertation, when the candidate typically struggles to interpret and make meaning of the results, especially if the study yielded negative findings. During the advisement process, of course, advisers work very closely with the candidate and may become invested in achieving a successful outcome. In such instances, in addition to containing and addressing the students' emotions, they may be struggling with their own feelings as well.

## STRATEGIES TO HELP STUDENTS ADDRESS THE CHALLENGES

A critical resource for helping doctoral students in coping with the aforementioned challenges is the faculty advisor. The best advisor generally is one who shares the student's topic of interest; has served on dissertation committees several times before taking on the role of a chair; and is familiar with the process, its pace, nuances, and possible barriers. Such a background enables an advisor to offer students clarity regarding expectations, time management, an understanding of where they are in the process, and help them anticipate what lies ahead.

As in practice interventions, for advisors to develop strategies that will best fit a particular advisee, an assessment of the latter is helpful. Specifically, it is useful to consider the student's motivation; commitment to the process and the topic; and ability to address the challenges intellectually, emotionally, and logistically (Gordon, 2003).

In addition to traditional teaching strategies used in professional education, such as integrating diverse modes of conveying knowledge to cater to different learning styles (Berger, 1996), using experiential learning, developing technology to enhance learning (Berger, Mullin, & Stein, 2008), and applying principles of adult learning, the following strategies can be beneficial in helping students with their dissertation.

First, to help candidates develop the necessary skills, compartmentalization and teaching in manageable incremental steps—while maintaining the connection to the big picture—support learning. Giving assignments that represent "mini-dissertations" and offering students opportunities to demonstrate their ability along the way are of utmost importance. For example, in a course on qualitative research, a first assignment may be focused on developing a research question that calls for a qualitative method. The assignment requires a scope-limited review of relevant empirical literature, the identification of gaps in the available knowledge, and the conceptualization of a research question designed to address one of the gaps. This exercise would be followed by a rationale about the significance of the question and for the use of a specific qualitative methodology to research it. The final step involves a clear articulation of the research approach to studying the question, informed by comments to the previous work. Such assignments allow students to develop a degree of comfort with what is involved in planning and conducting an independent project and to begin to hone their skills, the absence of which were identified as the greatest obstacle to successful completion of a dissertation (D'Andrea, 2002). Furthermore, the argument often is made that a student's course papers should lead to a literature review and preliminary plan for a dissertation. Some programs offer courses that require students to focus on their dissertation work through the development of a literature review and discussion of a pertinent research method in preparation for the dissertation. Proponents cite the process more prevalent in the health sciences (especially where the use of laboratories and equipment is required), where the dissertation is composed of a set of research papers, of which the candidate is a primary contributor. Opponents frequently emphasize the importance of using assignments written during courses as a platform from which a dissertation topic is developed. No evidence for the superiority of either of these models is currently available.

Skills achieved via these assignments can be strengthened further by opportunities to participate in research early on. For example, advisees may be offered a chance to take part in the advisor's research activities, such as recruitment of participants, collecting and analyzing data, so that when it comes to conducting their own dissertation study they already have familiarity and firsthand experience with conducting research in the field.

Second, a lot of practice is needed to help students acquire mastery of "translating" theoretical frameworks into a research agenda. One useful strategy is providing abundant opportunities for "toying" with concept-to-variable and the tenets of hypothesis development. For instance, an assignment in a course about issues and strategies for researching families might require each student to identify a theory about family development, dynamics, or therapy; identify two empirical articles that report studies informed by the theory; and lead a class discussion of the theory and its application as described in the two articles. Such assignments allow students to move gradually from "passive" to "active" implementation of theory as it informs research.

Also helpful in all phases of the process is offering relevant sections from previous successful proposals and dissertations as templates. For example, students can be presented with examples of focus of inquiry sections (with the authors' permission) relative to a diverse range of topics in order to allow them to capture the underlying thought process of a well-justified and conceptualized research question. Furthermore, students in advanced phases of their doctoral education (and recent graduates) may be invited as guest speakers to share their journey and hurdles they encountered, along with resources and practices that helped them.

To assist students in developing the necessary intellectual flexibility for the theory–research connection, several approaches can be used. One would involve guiding them to look at the question that interests them through the lens of diverse theoretical perspectives. Thus, a student interested in the experience with service providers of previously abused minority women was asked to evaluate a research approach informed by several relevant conceptual frameworks, such as standpoints theory and postmodernistic feminism, before she chose a specific theory to use in her study.

Encouraging students to identify and contact key people in their field of interest has repeatedly proved to be a fruitful way to gain access to current knowledge (such as unpublished manuscripts), as well as broadening networking opportunities with others interested in similar topics. Candidates often are apprehensive about approaching established scholars whom they perceive as "bigger than life." When asked who has emerged from their review of relevant literature as dominant figures in their field of interest, and whether they contacted these individuals, students provide the typical response that they would not know what to ask and that they are certain that such "important" people would not bother to respond. More than one candidate who followed the encouragement to contact a leader in their field of interest reported being surprised at receiving an instant, favorable, and supportive response—with helpful information about recent publications, improved instruments, and updates on new developments.

In addition to students receiving direct help from their advisor/mentor, it is also frequently useful for students to be referred to available "hidden" resources, where they can find platforms to share their struggles and seek advice. For example, the Society for Social Work Research has a doctoral student center that offers practical tips about a wide and diverse range of advice about issues relevant to students with families and online support to strategies for self care.

Using peer support has been reported as helpful, as well (Johnson & Conyers, 2001), especially in the early phases of the dissertation (Burnett, 1999). Such support can be received from a cohort or online and may help mitigate the feeling of loneliness, provide role models, create a pool of ideas when students feel "stuck," serve as a sounding board, provide a structure, and assist in setting realistic goals. Peer support is particularly helpful for international doctoral students, who compose 18.5% of full-time and 3.3% of part-time students taking courses (CSWE, 2012). They can benefit from feedback from those whose native language is English regarding their writing, learn about cultural norms of the host country, and gain a family-like experience. However, such peer support is not necessarily ideal for all. Some decline to participate in a regular peer support group because they already are struggling with family and employment responsibilities and prefer to use the remaining limited time for actual work on the dissertation.

On a smaller scale, advisees who appear to be compatible routinely are "matched" for creating their own support dyad. Matching students working on their dissertation with others with similar interests can offer practical support, such as reviewing each other's interview transcriptions and identifying resources. For example, a student who was in the middle stages of interviewing mothers of children who were unexpectedly born with a developmental disability was paired with a student who was interviewing home health aides about their experiences. Although the topics were different, the challenges involved in recruitment, engagement, and collecting data in qualitative research allowed the two students to consult, offer one another practical help, and lend a friendly ear when the process became stressful. The aforementioned strategies are best implemented in the context of developing a relationship with students in which the teacher's role emphasizes interaction and mentoring of academic professionals in the making and of helping to remove psychological blocks and offering consistent support (Baird, 1992).

In addition to the advisement process, support from members of the committee, the department, and the institution also is necessary. Institutional supports that have been recommended in a national PhD Completion Project include hosting of dissertation "boot camps," retreats, and workshops to help enhance students' scholarly abilities; recognizing outstanding dissertations; offering training for advisors to improve their skills; providing opportunities for the development of doctoral student communities; and fostering a collegial research environment (Council of Graduate Schools, 2008). In addition, the institution of structures for monitoring progress has been recommended (Strachan, Murray, & Grierson, 2004). Also helpful is providing departmental support for students to present at conferences and encouraging them to submit articles so that when they get to the stage of dissertation development they have had some understanding of and engagement in the process of scholarly writing.

## SUMMARY AND CONCLUSIONS

Although the ideas discussed in this article are rooted in the author's many years of experience in social work doctoral education, they are based on some anecdotal and impressionistic data as well. Systematic research now is needed to evaluate the effectiveness of these and other strategies from the perspectives of instructors, mentors and advisors, and graduates, as well as students currently in various phases of the process. Such research will allow social work doctoral programs to develop a more nuanced understanding of what works and for whom, potentially enhancing the quality of the experience and increasing both the pace and prevalence of successful graduation.

## ACKNOWLEDGMENTS

I thank Dr. Judy Fenster of Adelphi University School of Social Work for inspiring the writing of this article and Dr. Ellen Rosenberg for commenting on a previous version.

## REFERENCES

Aitchison, C. (2009). Writing groups for doctoral education. *Studies in Higher Education, 34*, 905–916. doi:10.1080/03075070902785580

Anastas, J. W., & Kuerbis, A. N. (2009). Doctoral education in social work: What we know and what we need to know. *Social Work, 54*, 71–81. doi:10.1093/sw/54.1.71

Anderson, L. W., & Krathwohl, D. R. (Eds.). (2001). *A taxonomy for learning, teaching and assessing: A revision of Bloom's taxonomy of educational objective.* New York, NY: Longman.

Baird, L. L. (1992, April). *The stages of the doctoral career: Socialization and its consequences.* Paper presented at the annual meeting of the American Educational Research Association, San Francisco, CA.

Berger, R. (1996). A comparative analysis of different methods of teaching group work. *Social Work with Groups, 19,* 79–89. doi:10.1300/J009v19n01_07

Berger, R. (2010). EBP: Practitioners in search of evidence. *Journal of Social Work, 10,* 175–191. doi:10.1177/1468017310363640

Berger, R., Mullin, J., & Stein, L. (2008). Videoconferencing: A viable teaching strategy for social work education? *Social Work Education, 27,* 1–12. doi:10.1080/02615470802308625

Bloom, B. S. (Ed.). (1956). *Taxonomy of educational objectives: The classification of educational goals.* London, UK: Longmans.

Burnett, P. C. (1999). The supervision of doctoral dissertations using a collaborative cohort model. *Counselor Education & Supervision, 39,* 46–52. doi:10.1002/j.1556-6978.1999.tb01789.x

Council of Graduate Schools. (2008). *Ph.D. completion project.* Retrieved from http://www.phdcompletion.org

Council of Social Work Education. (2008). *2008 educational policy and accreditation standards.* Washington, DC: Author. Retrieved from http://www.cswe.org/File.aspx

Council on Social Work Education. (2012). *Statistics on social work education in the United States.* Retrieved from http://www.cswe.org/File.aspx?id=68977

D'Andrea, L. M. (2002). Obstacles to completion of the doctoral degree in colleges of education: The professors' perspective. *Educational Research Quarterly, 25*(3), 42–58.

Di Pierro, M. (2007). Excellence in doctoral education: Defining best practices. *College Student Journal, 41,* 368–375.

Ferguson, C. (2002). Using the revised taxonomy to plan and deliver team-taught integrated, thematic units. *Theory into Practice, 41,* 238–243. doi:10.1207/s15430421tip4104_6

Gordon, P. J. (2003). Advising to avoid or to cope with dissertation hang-ups. *Academy of Management Learning & Education, 2,* 181–187. doi:10.5465/AMLE.2003.9901674

Jenson, J. M. (2008). Enhancing research capacity and knowledge development through social work doctoral education. *Social Work Research, 32,* 3–5. doi:10.1093/swr/32.1.3

Johnson, R. W., & Conyers, L. M. (2001). Surviving the doctoral dissertation: A solution-focused approach. *Journal of College Counseling, 4,* 77–80. doi:10.1002/j.2161-1882.2001.tb00185.x

Kornbeck, J. (2007). Social work academics as Humboldtian researcher-educators: Discussion of a survey of staff profiles from schools in Denmark, England and Germany. *Social Work Education, 26,* 86–100. doi:10.1080/02615470601036591

Krathwohl, D. R. (2002). A revision of bloom's taxonomy: An overview. *Theory into Practice, 41,* 212–218. doi:10.1207/s15430421tip4104_2

Liechty, J. M., Liao, M., & Schull, C. (2009). Facilitating dissertation completion and success among doctoral students in social work. *Journal of Social Work Education, 45,* 481–497. doi:10.5175/JSWE.2009.200800091

Mays, T. L., & Smith, B. (2009). Navigating the doctoral journey. *Journal of Hospital Librarianship*, *9*, 345–361. doi:10.1080/15323260903250411.

Society of College National and University Libraries. (2007). *Seven pillars model for information literacy*. Retrieved from http://www.sconul.ac.uk/groups/information_literacy/sp/model.html

Spillett, M. A., & Moisiewicz, K. A. (2004). Cheerleader, coach, counselor or critic: Support and challenge roles of the dissertation. *College Student Journal*, *38*, 246–256.

Spring, H. (2010). Theories of learning: Models of good practice for evidence-based information skills teaching. *Health Information & Libraries Journal*, *27*, 327–331. doi:10.1111/j.1471-1842.2010.00911.x

Stoesz, D., Karger, H. J., & Carrilio, T. (2010). *A dream deferred*. New Brunswick, NJ: Transaction Publishers.

Strachan, R., Murray, R., & Grierson, H. (2004). A web-based tool for dissertation writing. *British Journal of Educational Technology*, *35*, 369–375. doi:10.1111/j.0007-1013.2004.00395.x

Sussman, T., Stoddart, K., & Gorman, E. (2004). Reconciling the congruent and contrasting roles of social work teacher, student and practitioner: An experiential account of three doctoral students. *Journal of Teaching in Social Work*, *24*, 161–179. doi:10.1300/J067v24n01_10

Wineburg, S., & Schneider, J. (2010). Was Bloom's taxonomy pointed in the wrong direction? *Phi Delta Kappan*, *91*, 56–61. doi:10.1177/003172171009100412

# Guiding Social Work Doctoral Graduates Through Scholarly Publications and Presentations

CYNTHIA L. GRANT

*Arapahoe Douglas Mental Health Network, Englewood, Colorado, USA*
*School of Education and Human Development, University of Colorado-Denver,*
*Denver, Colorado, USA*

DANIEL R. TOMAL

*Department of Educational Leadership, Concordia University Chicago,*
*River Forest, Illinois, USA*

*Disseminating the work of social work doctoral graduates aligns with the Council on Social Work Education's National Statement on Research Integrity in Social Work publication practices and the National Association of Social Workers Code of Ethics. Publications and presentations are essential to their future success, yet little support is provided to social work doctoral graduates by programs that are not affiliated with research universities. This article fills a gap in the literature by offering faculty a clear guide on how to engage graduates in the scholarly dissemination of their advanced practice skills and dissertation research through publications and presentations.*

## BACKGROUND

The vast majority of doctoral social work graduates undoubtedly will continue to advance their careers following graduation. One of the most universally effective ways to achieve this goal is through scholarly publications and presentations. Although it may be expected that a PhD graduate who attended a research intensive institution (while receiving dissertation research financial support in the form of tuition waivers, research assistantships or fellowships) will engage in these endeavors, we believe the same expectations should exist for all doctoral social work graduates. In fact, the Council of Social Work Education (CSWE) convened a Doctor of Social Work (DSW) task force in 2011 and outlined key elements of the DSW degree, including a guideline that each student should "engage in active practice based research and disseminate findings through presentations and publications" (Rittner, Holmes, & Edwards, 2011, p. 11). Similarly, national initiatives to address the "science of social work," as well as the need to communicate new knowledge to others, have been published elsewhere in relation to the importance of scholarly publication within the profession (Brekke, 2012; Fong, 2013).

The Group for the Advancement of Doctoral Education (GADE) Task Force on Quality Guidelines recommends that doctoral programs should encourage students to present at least twice and to have completed two or three sole or co-authored articles in peer-reviewed journals prior to graduation (Harrington, Petr, Black, & Cunningham-Williams, 2013). Research universities often fund doctoral education for candidates and engage in pedagogical practices that allow for these goals to more easily be achieved. Programs that use mentoring models and provide financial support for scholarly development are commended for their provision of supports to cultivate a doctoral-level scholar. Yet the proliferation of professional practice doctoral programs in the United States and abroad (e.g., DSW programs); the plethora of social work programs that are not focused on research; the popularity of part-time, clinically focused PhD programs (e.g., Smith College, the Institute for Clinical Social Work); and the more recent emergence of online, for-profit doctoral degree programs in social work (e.g., Capella University and Walden University) present a quandary. Many of these programs offer exceptional advanced clinical practice and program development training but offer little support or guidance to doctoral students on how to publish and present both as a student and upon graduation.

Doctoral degree programs in social work are not accredited by the CSWE, and therefore uniform comprehensive data on doctoral education in social work is difficult to gather. GADE is commonly recognized in the field as the best source of information. As of January 2014, there were 74 institutional members of GADE in the United States and an additional nine international institutions (www.gadephd.org). Yet the GADE membership directory is incomplete. Based on information available online, there appears to be at least one additional ground-based degree program (Aurora University) and two online institutions (Capella University and Walden University) in the United States offering the DSW that are not listed in the GADE directory. Additional DSW programs are scheduled to start at Tulane University, St. Catherine University–the University of St. Thomas, and the

**TABLE 1** Doctor of Social Work Programs

| University | Location |
| --- | --- |
| Aurora University | Aurora, Illinois, USA |
| Capella University | Online |
| Cardiff University | Cardiff, Wales, UK |
| Rutgers University | New Brunswick, New Jersey, USA |
| St. Catherine University–University of St. Thomas[a] | St. Paul, Minnesota, USA |
| Tulane University[a] | New Orleans, Louisiana, USA |
| University of Dundee | Dundee, Scotland, UK |
| University of Pennsylvania | Philadelphia, Pennsylvania, USA |
| University of Portsmouth | Portsmouth, England, UK |
| University of Southern California[b] | Online |
| University of Sussex | Brighton, England, UK |
| University of Sydney | Sydney, Australia |
| University of Tennessee | Knoxville, Tennessee, USA |
| Walden University | Online |

[a]Programs scheduled to begin in August 2014. [b]Program scheduled to begin in 2015.

University of Southern California. An informal web search identified dozens of international ground-based PhD in Social Work programs and four international universities offering the DSW that are not listed in the GADE member directory. Table 1 includes a list of known English-speaking DSW programs, only three of which are listed in the GADE directory (Rutgers University, University of Pennsylvania, and the University of Tennessee–Knoxville).

In total, there are more than 100 institutions worldwide that offer a doctoral-level degree in social work. Programs offering doctoral degrees in the United States are classified as doctorate-granting research universities with very high research activity (RU/VH), high research activity, and as doctoral/research universities, based on the Carnegie Foundation Basic Classification framework (McCormick & Zhao, 2005). Very high research activities are indicative of greater expenditures on research and faculty whose primary responsibility is to engage in research (vs. instruction or public service) (Carnegie Foundation, 2010). These programs often offer tuition funding, fellowships, and/or research assistantships to doctoral students engaged in faculty sponsored research. Of the 74 U.S.-based doctoral social work programs identified in the GADE directory, 56.7% ($n = 42$) are offered at institutions classified as RU/VH universities. As such, faculty teaching at the remaining 43.3% of GADE member institutions (plus others not listed in their directory) may have limited resources available to social work doctoral candidates for mentoring research activity, publication, and presentation.

In their most recent 2012 statistical report, CSWE published a survey of doctoral programs in the United States based on responses from 62 GADE member institutions out of a possible 73 members during the year that data were collected. Almost all survey data (96.8%, $n = 60$) were derived from PhD-granting institutions. There were 2,428 students enrolled in these

62 reporting doctoral social work programs in the 2011–2012 academic year. Similar to years past, CSWE reported that 307 students in 2012 received their doctoral degree in social work, with 97.1% ($n = 298$) of the reported degrees being the PhD. The 2012 response rate to this survey, however, was 84.9% ($n = 62$) and included only institutions that were members of GADE. Thus, one can safely assume that the actual numbers of doctoral graduates were even higher given that there were additional institutions not included in the study sample.

The information portal for prospective students posted on the GADE website describes many career paths for doctoral-degree holding social workers (see http://gadephd.org). Positions include faculty-research, administration, advanced practice careers, and public policy positions. From the 2012 GADE member survey data, CSWE (2013) reported the following statistics on the employment of PhD graduates, shown in Table 2.

A number of limitations are present in these data. CSWE collected information only from GADE member institutions, which excluded for-profit universities and most of the International DSW advanced practice doctorate programs. As a result, these statistics are heavily weighted toward research-focused PhDs and may not fully capture the full range of doctorates in the profession. In addition, as one can see, the employment status of 17.3% of graduates is unknown. According to Dr. Dorothy Kagehiro (personal communication, January 9, 2014), Research Associate at CSWE, "programs have difficulty tracking what happens to their graduates," and CSWE does not disaggregate postgraduation items based on the type of degree. In addition,

**TABLE 2** CSWE Report of 2013 Doctoral Graduate Employment Status*

| Employment status | No. | % |
|---|---|---|
| Tenure-line faculty position in CSWE-accredited program | 143 | 35.2 |
| Academic research position | 30 | 7.4 |
| Nonacademic administrative position | 27 | 6.7 |
| Non–tenure-line faculty position in CSWE-accredited program | 26 | 6.4 |
| Postdoctoral fellow | 25 | 6.2 |
| Private clinical practice | 23 | 5.7 |
| Academic administrative position | 13 | 3.2 |
| Nonacademic research position | 12 | 3.0 |
| Faculty position in a program not accredited by CSWE | 12 | 3.0 |
| Consulting position | 8 | 2.0 |
| Other | 36 | 8.9 |
| Not employed | 13 | 3.2 |
| Unknown | 38 | 9.4 |
| Total doctoral graduates | 406 | |
| Programs reporting | 57 | |

*Most recent data available at time of publication.

© 2013 Council on Social Work Education. Reproduced by permission of the Council on Social Work Education. Permission to reuse must be obtained from the rightsholder.

there is no known database on the number of publications or presentations of doctoral-degree-holding social work graduates, which makes it even more difficult for the profession to highlight the frequency of scholarly work produced by its doctoral graduates. Regardless of these gaps, guidelines published by a GADE Task Force on Quality Guidelines outlined the goals, core expertise, and skills expected of PhD graduates—including the importance of disseminating their dissertation findings.

The purpose of this article is to offer guidance for faculty working with doctoral students on how to teach candidates to engage in scholarly dissemination of their dissertation research through publications and presentations. Given the demands on full-time faculty to pursue their own scholarship, coupled with the need to attend to currently enrolled doctoral candidates, it is understandable that they may not have time or resources to continue to mentor graduates after they have earned their degree. Nonetheless, this article can be shared with doctoral candidates to offer clear steps to take to meet the expectations of the National Association of Social Workers (NASW; 2008) Code of Ethics that social workers be involved in advancing the integrity of the profession through publications and presentations.

This article draws from a collection of the authors' experiences in higher education, serving on dissertation committees, as well as a PhD in social work graduate from an institution that did not offer research intensive resources, or familiarity with the "publish or perish" expectation placed on individuals who secure employment in tenure-track academic positions. Such expectations further justify the need to help new doctoral graduates succeed in the dissemination of their dissertation findings.

## PUBLISHING THE DISSERTATION

There are many advantages to sharing one's work—both initially as a completed dissertation available in a library or online databases, and taking the dissemination of the dissertation findings one step further with publications or presentations. As faculty members are keenly aware, some of these benefits include the chance to further one's career (Kelsky, 2011), to advance the professional field, gain personal satisfaction, assist other scholars, and build one's reputation as a subject expert (Wood, 2014). Publications and presentations inevitably help graduates who take on academic positions, and are becoming more respected in practice. Disseminating one's work shows initiative and aligns with the CSWE (2006) National Statement on Research Integrity in Social Work publication practices.

Prior to making a decision about publishing or presenting their work, faculty should help doctoral candidates and graduates identify the intended goals of dissemination. Articles are published to influence practitioners, to inform policymakers, to highlight research methods used in the field, and to share the discovery of new knowledge. Faculty should consider whether the publication and presentation goals of the doctoral candidate align with the future career aspirations of the graduate whether it is to secure an academic appointment or to help achieve nonacademic career goals or building one's reputation as a content expert. Each of these goals may suggest a different audience for publication and presentation.

At a minimum, all PhD and DSW graduates should publish their dissertation. The doctoral chairperson often is the point person to guide the new graduate on how to copyright the dissertation, which allows ownership of the material and compensation for infringement. The complexities of copyright laws are beyond the scope of this article (especially with dissertations involving sponsored research; Crews, 2013). Graduates may have their work copyrighted directly through the U.S. Copyright Office at eCo.com, or may use ProQuest Dissertations and Theses/UMI, which will complete the service for them. The copyright is owned by the graduate, not UMI.

Many graduates authorize publication of the dissertation in its original form using UMI Dissertation Publishing, which is a part of ProQuest Dissertations and Theses (PQDT). PQDT is accessible at more than 3,000 libraries worldwide. The PQDT/UMI collection noted is a repository of dissertations and theses. Publication with PQDT/UMI allows graduates to electronically submit their dissertations for open access or traditional publishing. There is debate among publishers and academicians about the use of the Internet to publicly disseminate intellectual property online using open access (Djurkovic, 2014). Faculty can instruct graduates on what procedures are permitted and determine if the school may have a policy on these publishing practices.

*Traditional publishing* allows for PQDT/UMI to list the dissertation's availability through an electronic subscription database purchased by library affiliates. There currently are more than 2 million entries in the database (ProQuest, n.d.), and more than 22,000 dissertations or theses in the Social Sciences database are filed with a subject heading for social work. PQDT/UMI publication trends indicate a significant increase in the number of social work dissertations entered in the database over the past 30 years, as displayed in Figure 1.

All graduates who choose to publish their work with PQDT/UMI will have their dissertation registered in their name to certify authorship. A copy of the work also will be deposited in the Library of Congress. Publishing the dissertation will automatically provide a publication number so that the work can be referenced with a legitimate citation (instead of as an unpublished manuscript). There are fees associated with each of these services. Faculty should direct graduates to review the PQDT/UMI website for more details and for instructions on how to format the dissertation for publication and printing.

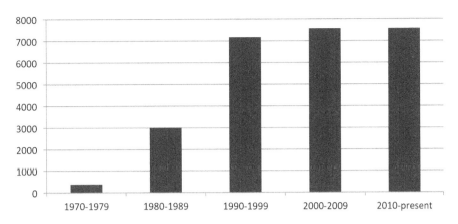

**FIGURE 1** PQDT/UMI social work dissertations and theses publications by date.

*Open access publishing* allows the dissertation to be accessible to the public in an electronic format available as a free download through PQDT Open. Some universities may require this publication format, especially if the dissertation was completed with support from federal funding. On the other hand, some institutions may prohibit or discourage open access publishing, especially if the research material is protected with respect to the study sample or study site. For graduates who choose to make their work available online at no charge to the public, the two most popular options currently are OpenThesis.org and Academia.edu. OpenThesis.org offers authors the opportunity to post their dissertation in a free and centralized online database. Faculty need to be aware of whether their institution has an account with OpenThesis.org to automatically publish the dissertation, or if graduates need to upload their work directly to the site. Similarly, Academia.edu is a popular platform for academics to share their research papers. The site allows users to electronically upload their dissertations (with associated keywords) that will link to Google searches of related information on the Internet. Academia.edu also tracks user analytics, such as how many times the dissertation was reviewed and how it is appearing in searches. Like other open source websites (e.g., Research Gate, PILOTS Database, Creative Commons), Academia.edu does not claim ownership rights to any of the materials posted on their site.

The dissertation is an ideal source for a new doctoral graduate to extract articles for publication under the guidance of experienced faculty. One dissertation study may, in fact, generate several articles and provide a foundation for other research studies associated with the original one. Faculty members therefore may need to direct new graduates to shift their view of the dissertation from a single, cohesive document to one that can be separated out for the purpose of publication.

## GUIDING GRADUATES ON THE TYPES OF PUBLICATIONS

Many social work graduates from non-RU/VH institutions do not submit their dissertation research findings for scholarly publication—beyond traditional or open access publication of the dissertation. There are a number of reasons that may contribute to this reality, including the demands of a new job, an experience of fatigue and loss of interest in the research topic, a lack of mentoring on the submission process, and the fear of rejection. Rejection rates for peer-reviewed journals range from 50% to more than 90% (Wagner, 2006), although Hopps and Morris (2007) reported that the average rejection rate for social work journals is lower than for other professions. Faculty members therefore should guide candidates in how to publish and present the dissertation beyond filing the document in its original form. Options include giving presentations; workshops; consulting; and publishing through articles, trade magazines, books, or private companies interested in the work. The most expected and recommended approach to disseminate one's work is through scholarly publication.

Scholarly publications are *peer reviewed* (also known as refereed). Although faculty is familiar with this practice, it may be helpful to clarify the process with graduates considering submission of a manuscript. When an article is submitted to a peer-reviewed journal, the editor typically distributes the manuscript to other scholars in the field to gather their opinion of the quality of the scholarship, the relevance to the professional field of practice, and appropriateness for the journal. There are many options available for publication in the field and across disciplines. Hence, thinking about where to publish elements of the dissertation may be an overwhelming experience for many new graduates.

One may wish to ascertain the ranking of a journal when considering where to submit a manuscript. One measure of a journal's ranking is the impact factor, which measures the number of times a journal article has been cited in a year as documented in Google Scholar (i.e., "Cited by #") or by the Journal Citation Report Social Science edition published by Thomson Reuters. For the most up-to-date list of journal rankings, based on impact scores and use, authors can review the Scientific Journal Ranking at www.scimagojr.com/journalrank. There are 61 U.S. and international journals listed in this database using a subject area search for "social sciences" and the subject category of "social work." The three highest ranking journals in the field of social work are currently from the United Kingdom: *Child Development; Journal of Marriage and Family*; and *Trauma, Violence, and Abuse*. In addition, Leung and Cheung (2013) of the University of Houston Graduate School of Social Work maintain an up-to-date journal database of social work manuscript submission information and impact factors (including those in the 2012 Journal Citation Report; University of Houston, n.d.). Faculty should share these resources with doctoral graduates.

Although a peer-reviewed journal that publishes quantitative, empirically based studies is usually the highest ranked, there is a cadre of alternative forms of scholarship the graduate may consider for publication. A *trade publication* for a nonacademic audience is appropriate for topics that apply to the general population and to practitioners in the field. Magazines, newsletters, and blogs for a nonprofit organization offer a way for new graduates to establish themselves in the field and with a target community. These generally are written in a more natural, conversational tone and rarely contain references or statistical tables. These manuscripts can be easy to write and may serve as a confidence booster to the graduate with little or no publication experience. Alternatively, trade publications may be a good choice of publication for scholars who are established in their field of expertise. Some examples of such publications include *The New Social Worker, NASW News, Social Work Today Magazine*, www.socialworknews.net, a newsletter for an agency, or a practitioner website.

*Review articles* are a good way for doctoral graduates to make use of the literature covered typically in Chapter 2 of the dissertation. They can include not only a synthesis of articles related to a topic but also the critical analysis, controversies, and gaps in the existing research. Much of the material in such articles is highly consistent with the tenants of a well-written dissertation literature review. Examples can readily be found in social work library database searches by adding the word "review" to a topic query, such as the article "Recovery in Severe Mental Illness: A Literature Review of Recovery Measures" by Scheyett, DeLuca, and Morgan published in the 2013 volume of *Social Work Research*.

*Theoretical articles* are written based on a person's thoughts. These articles may review an existing theory, offer a new theoretical approach to a topic, or highlight an idea for future research. Theoretical perspectives are greatly valued in academia, and some authors prefer this type of scholarly publication so that their opinions can be shared publicly. A seminal example of this type of article is "The Strengths Perspective in Social Work Practice: Extensions and Cautions" by Dennis Saleebey (1996).

*Practice articles* offer descriptions or case examples of approaches used in professional practice. Rather than coming from a research perspective, manuscripts are built from practice wisdom and the expertise of the authors, based on their experiences in the field. This article is one example of such a publication. Like theoretical articles, these pieces offer ideas for future research and can be a good fit for clinical PhD or DSW program graduates. The *Clinical Social Work Journal* and the *Journal of Social Work Practice* are leaders in the field for publishing practice articles.

Unlike the aforementioned publication types, *research articles* provide empirical evidence via data that were collected and analyzed by the researcher. They are not based on one's thoughts, opinions, or a review of others' works but detail an original, scholarly, research-based contribution to the field. Almost all social work journals include research-based manuscripts. Such submissions may derive from quantitative, qualitative, or mixed methods studies. In addition, some periodicals are specifically geared toward evidence-based practices, participatory action research, or program evaluation methods. These articles frequently are considered the most competitive of scholarly opportunities and may have the greatest impact on the graduate's reputation as a scholar in academia. Examples of empirical articles can be found throughout most journals, including *Social Work, Social Service Review, British Journal of Social Work, Health & Social Work, Research on Social Work Practice*, and the *Journal of Social Service Research*.

## GUIDING GRADUATES ON THE PUBLICATION PROCESS

Graduates with limited experience in publication submission need to be coached on how to identify suitable sources for publication. Faculty should encourage graduates not to limit themselves to one discipline. Many journals are multidisciplinary; research and subject topic journals encourage and accept submissions across many professions. Seasoned faculty members can offer expertise on how to target a journal submission for publication. The need for authors to tailor writing and publication style for each journal and the ethical requirement that manuscripts be reviewed only by one journal at a time make it imperative that new authors select the most relevant journal in order to increase their chance for publication success.

Although there have been some efforts in the field of social work to provide guidance on how to choose a journal for manuscript submission (see the Society for Social Work Research Presidential Task Force on Publications Bulletin Board at http://sswrptfp.wordpress.com/), choosing where to submit one's work remains a process that each graduate must learn to navigate. Those who submit may have to wait up to a year to find out that their paper has been rejected, and they thus need to find another publisher. However, with mentored guidance from senior faculty, the graduates can learn how the carefully tailored selection of a journal will result in a greater likelihood of having the article accepted for publication.

Faculty may want to ensure that new authors are aware of some of the statistics associated with a publication when choosing where to submit. These features typically include the subscription rate, type of readers, acceptance rate, whether it is refereed, length of time for a decision, submission requirements, and length of runway before publishing after acceptance. One of the most important of these features is the acceptance rate. Journal acceptance rates can range from 1% to 50% (Wagner, 2006). Some of the more prestigious and competitive first-tier journals, such as *Qualitative Inquiry* and the *Journal of Teaching in Social Work*, have acceptance rates at the lowest levels of less than 10% (Walker, 2010). However, graduates need to understand that acceptance rates for a publication are not always the same at any given time and may vary, depending on the backlog of articles, which can range from a few months to a few years. An editor-in-chief may invite submissions in the form of a Call for Papers and may be more likely to accept a manuscript if the topic is related to the preselected focus, such as a special issue. (In the case of this article, for example, the authors responded to a call for papers for a special issue exclusively on doctoral education.)

New authors may not be aware that most peer-reviewed journals have websites to explain their submission process. Once a potential source is identified, the doctoral graduate should go to the website to determine whether the journal is a good fit with respect to the mission of the publication, style, and expectations. (The Society for Social Work Research Presidential Task Force on Publications, 2008, recommended that all publishers of social work journals should have publicly available information on the specific requirements of their journal.) Most professional periodicals provide instructions to authors, which is an outline of the guidelines and expectations for manuscript submissions. For example, the journal *Social Work* has an Information for Authors page that includes the history of the publication, topics of interest, desired length of articles, types of articles accepted, and a link to the editor's formatting requirements. Journal editors generally will also include writing guidelines with regard to spacing, margin settings, headings, subheadings, references, and formatting for figures and tables. In ideal situations, the journal will include a recommended checklist for authors to guide the process (Holosko, 2006).

Faculty may need to explain the blind review process used by most refereed journals. Once the editor-in-chief receives a manuscript submission, the author's name and organizational affiliation are removed, and the manuscript is sent to two or three undisclosed peer reviewers, without identifying information. Reviewers are given the submitted manuscript, an evaluation form, and a date when the reviewed manuscript is to be returned to the editor. Most manuscript evaluation forms will have several closed-ended questions with a Likert-style scale, a rubric, and open-ended questions. Some of the typical closed-ended questions include the following:

- Is the manuscript scholarly?
- Is the content specifically relevant to the journal's audience?
- Is the manuscript well organized and clearly written?
- Are the contents and references accurate and current?
- Are the format and structural mechanics clear?
- Is the manuscript easy to read and does it hold interest?
- Is the length appropriate for the journal?
- Are the conclusions relevant and clearly drawn?
- Do the reference citations conform to publication style?

- Are the literature review and methodology sections adequate?
- Does the manuscript represent a contribution to the field?

The evaluation form may also have one or more open-ended questions that allow the reviewers to include specific comments about the article. In some cases, the editor shares these comments (anonymously) with the author. Such feedback can be useful for future submissions or revision of the article. Typical open-ended questions include information regarding the strength of the manuscript and areas in need of improvement. Options for reviewers may include accept, accept pending minor revisions, option to resubmit with major revisions, or reject. The turnaround time for a decision may be as little as two to four months but can take much longer at first-tier journals. It is imperative for faculty to explain and prepare new authors for the fact that it is very rare for editors to accept an article without revisions. Faculty should coach graduates that a resubmission request is often a good sign that the manuscript may have a better chance of being accepted during the second review.

Social work faculty need to guide graduates on how to make the transition from dissertation writing to publication. New authors must be aware that journal articles are written for journal readership. The purpose of a journal article is not to convince a dissertation committee of the soundness of a research study, or to demonstrate doctoral competency in research methods, but rather to offer information to an audience of peers on what has been found and why it matters to the field (Grant & Tomal, 2013). Some graduates will try to convert the entire dissertation into a 15- to 20-page journal article. This is possible, as there are similarities in the organization of the five-chapter model dissertation and a typical research article. Each will have an abstract, an introduction, a review of the literature, a section on research methods, results, and a discussion. Dissertations designed by the committee as "with distinction" may be the most likely to achieve success with this option. However, the challenges of compressing a dissertation into one article are great and may not sit well with reviewers. Graduates who make this attempt face significant challenges in regard to the content, format, and length of converting the dissertation to a single article. For example, one may find that overinterpretation of results is a common problem with authors who attempt to transfer a dissertation in its entirety to a journal article (Thomas & Skinner, 2012). Recommended reference texts for beginning social work scholars include *The Columbia Guide to Social Work Writing* (Green & Simon, 2012) and *Professional Writing for Social Work Practice* (Weisman & Zornado, 2012).

Social work faculty supervising the dissertation may want to consider coauthoring an article with the recent graduate. An experienced co-author may help the new graduate develop a paper that is more likely to be accepted. Coauthoring also offers a way for the new scholar to give back to the chairperson for his or her contributions to the dissertation process and is an excellent opportunity for tenure-track faculty to highlight their involvement with emerging doctoral scholars.

## PRESENTING THE DISSERTATION AT CONFERENCES

Although publication of the dissertation is a valuable way to disseminate findings to the public, there is also great value for graduates to present their dissertation research at a conference, workshop, or colloquium. Conference presentations, moreover, are one way for social workers to "promote respect for the value, integrity, and competence of the social work profession," as called for in Standard 5.01 of the NASW (2008) Code of Ethics. Conference presentations offer exigent networking benefits for the new graduate and may have higher acceptance rates (in comparison to peer-reviewed journals). Nevertheless, in recent years some conferences have become as competitive as journals. For example, the 2013 SSWR annual conference had a 36% acceptance rate (E. Uehara, personal communication, June 27, 2014), and the *Journal of the Society for Social Work and Research* had an identical 36% acceptance rate during the same year (D. Wyant, personal communication, June 25, 2014).

National or regional meetings of professional organizations such as NASW, CSWE, and SSWR often post a call for proposals in advance of their conferences. Faculty should encourage social work graduates to be on appropriate e-mail listservs and to join organizations that are consistent with their specialization. Doctoral scholars should review trade publications and journals and check websites regularly for request for proposals (known as RFPs) in their areas of interest. Examples of such organizations include The School Social Work Association of America, The Association of Traumatic Stress Specialists, Clinical Social Work Association, and the Society for Leadership in Health Care. Submission deadlines usually are many months in advance of a conference, so it is important for doctoral candidates to review presentation guidelines prior to graduation.

Conference proposal requirements vary greatly. Some conferences require only a paragraph or two describing what will be presented; others require online submission of a completed paper of significant substance with American Psychological Association–formatted references. Faculty can review the proposal requirements carefully with doctoral candidates and new graduates to ensure the submitted presentation meets the theme of the conference, the format and criteria for the specific presentation, and the conference's overall objectives. In most cases conference organizers review a proposal submission anonymously and a decision is made fairly quickly.

Conference presentations take on multiple formats, each of which will have their own policies and guidelines. The least preparation (and easiest

way to gain entry) might include "lightning sessions" and poster presentations. On the other end of the spectrum, research paper presentations with
proceedings deposited into the organization's repository of papers represent a more advanced and more competitive opportunity. Faculty members
who have experience attending the conference where a doctoral graduate
is applying may be able to offer guidance on how to choose the type of
session to submit for a presentation.

*Lightning sessions* or *demonstrations* allow presenters a very short time
(often just 10–20 min) to present findings or ideas to an audience. The
Ontario Association of Social Workers and some state-level social work
chapter organizations offer such types of sessions. Presenters are grouped
together around similar topics and may use multimedia to show their work,
idea, or product. *Poster presentations* utilize a bulletin board display (often
with accompanying handouts) to discuss a completed research project or
one that is still under way. This forum allows presenters to actively engage
in informal discussions with other conference attendees and serves the function of allowing doctoral candidates and new graduates to network. Student
poster presentations currently are very popular at national social work organizational conferences and at university seminars. In addition, international
conferences such as the Joint World Conference on Social Work, Education
and Social Development have begun offering *e-poster presentations* that are
accessible to a wide audience online. *Roundtable discussions* situate small
groups for conversations that are intended to advance, enhance, or share
information about similar topics. Working papers often are distributed for discussion in the small group so that attendees may gather ideas and resources
to inform subsequent research or practice. All of the aforementioned sessions
offer an opportunity for dialogue, networking, and refinement of ideas.

A *panel discussion* usually involves four or five invited speakers (sometimes proposed by the panelists themselves) who share a time slot to discuss
similar issues. Panelists typically are seated in front of an audience that will
also engage in the presentation. *Special interest groups* (SIGs) involve short
meetings (or a minisession) of individuals who gather for a similar purpose of discussion. SIGs may sponsor roundtables or panel discussions and
provide a chance for scholars to introduce themselves to an organization
and to get to know others interested in a specific field of inquiry. SSWR,
the European Conference for Social Work, and the Association of Oncology
Social Workers all offer SIG sessions. Faculty who belong to a SIG may want
to invite graduates with similar interests to join them.

*Paper sessions* offer an occasion for authors to present their work-in-
progress. Presenters may be thematically grouped together for 15- to 30-min
presentations of each of their papers, or present alone for up to an hour.
When a group of colleagues present separate papers on a common topic or
theme, this is usually referred to as a colloquium. Although all conferences
typically have paper sessions, research colloquia and workshops tend to be

more common at the university level as part of a lecture series. Paper presentations may have a respondent who will give commentary on the presenter's work. The presenter will then be given time to respond to the comments. These scholarly papers generally do not present research methods and findings, but rather offer theoretical or conceptual talking points on a topic of interest. Some DSW graduates may find that their dissertation topics are well suited for this type of presentation.

Like the research article published in a peer-reviewed journal, the most prestigious conference presentations usually are its *research paper* presentations. The demonstration of a research paper offers formal public introduction to the results of a quantitative, qualitative, mixed methods, participatory action research, or sometimes even a program evaluation study. The five-chapter model used for most social work dissertations is ideal for this type of offering. Research paper presentation allows the graduate to share findings more comprehensively than other conference formats might allow.

It is becoming more common today for conferences to be offered both virtually and in person, although there remains some ambivalence among members of the social work profession in terms of acceptance of the use of online learning for professional development. Some states (e.g., Illinois and Michigan) have begun to limit the number of continuing education units that social workers can earn online. *Virtual presentations* or online *webinars* deliver content via the Internet in a format that is more affordable and often more convenient for many professionals (Oualha & Matula, 2009). *Teleconferences* delivered over the phone are also still in use by agencies and professional organizations, including NASW. Such presentations can be synchronous (i.e., with participants and the presenter attending in real time) or asynchronous (i.e., prerecorded information that can be reviewed online at any time). Social Work Resource, NASW, the Australian Association of Social Workers, and the National Council for Behavioral Health are all organizations that regularly offer virtual webinars or conferences.

Some of the advantages of virtual conference presentations are the increased number of participants, an opportunity to engage individuals across cultures and geography, and the chance to reach those who are on the job and unable to afford or attend in person conferences (Young, 2009). Disadvantages include the lack of interactivity of participants (especially when there is a large number), a risk of participants leaving the session, and lack of technology skills among presenters. Nonetheless, this format for delivering a presentation is growing in quality and quantity in the field and is another scholarly option for disseminating one's work.

It is becoming more common for conference presenters to be asked to share their work in an online database associated with the conference or to submit papers to a journal affiliated with the sponsoring organization. In fact, Perron and colleagues (2011) found that 43% of SSWR conference presentations ultimately were published in a peer-reviewed journal at a later date regardless of the type of presentation. Social work organizations in the United States, Great Britain, and Australia all offer these opportunities. Interdisciplinary conferences also encourage uploading documents to their websites for public access.

## CONCLUSIONS

Faculty of both PhD and DSW programs are encouraged to work with social work doctoral candidates and graduates to lead them on how to present and publish from their dissertations in order to disseminate findings to the profession and society. Social science doctoral program candidates spend an average of 2 years working on their dissertation (Rudestam & Newton, 2007), but the guidance provided by faculty should not end with its completion. A doctoral faculty has an obligation to aid graduates in the distribution of newly acquired knowledge and to encourage them to market and network their strengths, expertise, and knowledge. Many postdoctoral scholars use their dissertation as a springboard for future research and employment. The dissertation topic of inquiry may set the stage for a research agenda that can be pursued in the field. Doctoral social work faculty should provide ongoing guidance to ensure that graduates know of the numerous possibilities for further scholarship and see mentoring of candidates and graduates as part of their pedagogical responsibility.

## REFERENCES

Brekke, J. (2012). Shaping a science of social work. *Research on Social Work Practice, 22,* 455–464. doi:10.1177/1049731512441263

Carnegie Foundation. (2010). *Carnegie Foundation methodology basic classifications.* Retrieved from http://classifications.carnegiefoundation.org/methodology/basic.php

Council on Social Work Education. (2006). *National statement on research integrity in social work.* Retrieved from http://www.cswe.org/cms/17157.aspx

Council on Social Work Education. (2013). *2012 statistics on social work education in the United States.* Retrieved from http://www.cswe.org/CentersInitiatives/DataStatistics/ProgramData.aspx

Crews, K. (2013). *Copyright and your dissertation or thesis: Ownership, fair use, and your rights and responsibilities.* Retrieved from http://www.proquest.com/assets/literature/services/copyright_dissthesis_ownership.pdf

Djurkovic, H. (2014). Debate: Open access in academic journal publishing. *Public Money and Management, 34,* 8–10. doi:10.1080/09540962.2014.865926

Fong, R. (2013). Framing doctoral education for a science of social work: Positioning students for the scientific career, promoting scholars for the academy, propagating scientists of the profession, and preparing stewards of the discipline. *Research on Social Work Practice*. Advance online publication. doi:10.1177/1049731513515055

Grant, C., & Tomal, D. (2013). *How to defend and finish your dissertation: Strategies to complete the professional practice doctorate*. Lantham, MA: Rowman & Littlefield Education.

Green, W., & Simon, B. (2012). *The Columbia guide to social work writing*. New York, NY: Columbia University Press.

Harrington, D., Petr, C., Black, B., & Cunningham-Williams, R. (2013). *Quality guidelines for PhD programs in social work. GADE Task Force on Quality Guidelines*. Retrieved from http://www.gadephd.org/LinkClick.aspx?fileticket=6RvhDyHRxQA%3D&tabid=84&portalid=0

Holosko, M. J. (2006). A suggested authors' checklist for submitting manuscripts to research on social work practice. *Research on Social Work Practice*, *16*, 449–454. doi:10.1177/1049731506288441

Hopps, J., & Morris, R. (Eds.). (2007). *Social work at the millennium: Critical reflections on the future of the profession*. New York, NY: The Free Press.

Kelsky, K. (2011, September 28). To: Professors; Re: Your advisees. *The Chronicle of Higher Education*. Retrieved from http://chronicle.com/article/To-Professors-Re-Your/129121/

Leung, P., & Cheung, M. (2013). *Journals in social work and related disciplines manuscript submission information*. Graduate College of Social Work, University of Houston. Retrieved from http://www.sw.uh.edu/_docs/cwep/journalsImpactFactorsHIndex.pdf

McCormick, A., & Zhao, C. (2005). Rethinking and reframing the Carnegie classification. *Change: The Magazine of Higher Learning*, *37*(5), 51–57. doi:10.3200/CHNG.37.5.51-57

National Association of Social Workers. (2008). *NASW code of ethics*. Washington, DC: Author.

Oualha, L., & Matula, T. (2009). The potential of online academic conferences to increase faculty interaction in a networked world. *European Journal of Management*, *9*(4), 185–188.

Perron, B., Taylor, H., Vaughn, M., Grogan-Kaylor, A., Ruffolo, M., & Spencer, M. (2011). From SSWR to peer-reviewed publication: How many live and how many die? *Research on Social Work Practice*, *21*, 594–598. doi:10.1177/1049731511402217

Proquest. (n.d.). *Proquest dissertations & theses database overview*. Retrieved from http://www.proquest.com/products-services/pqdt.html

Rittner, B., Holmes, J., & Edwards, R. (2011). *The doctorate in social work (DSW) degree: Emergence of a new practice doctorate*. Retrieved from http://www.cswe.org/File.aspx?id=59954

Rudestam, K., & Newton, R. (2007). *Surviving your dissertation: A comprehensive guide to content and process* (3rd ed.). Thousand Oaks, CA: Sage.

Saleebey, D. (1996). The strengths perspective in social work practice: Extensions and cautions. *Social Work*, *41*, 296–305.

Scheyett, A., DeLuca, J., & Morgan, C. (2013). Recovery in severe mental illnesses: A literature review of recovery measures. *Social Work Research*, *37*(3), 286–303. doi:10.1093/swr/svt018

Society for Social Work and Research Presidential Task Force on Publications. (2008). *Journal publication practices in social work*. Retrieved from http://www.sswr.org/PTFP%20final%20report%202008.pdf

Thomas, B., & Skinner, H. (2012). Dissertation to journal article: A systematic approach. *Educational Research International*, Article ID 862135, 11. doi:10.1155/2012/862135

University of Houston. (n.d.). *National Title IV-E website*. Retrieved from http://www.sw.uh.edu/community/cwep/title-iv-e/index.php .

Wagner, E. (2006). Ethics: What is it for? *Nature*. doi:10.1038/nature04990

Walker, J. (2010). *Journal acceptance rates*. Retrieved from http://guides.library.uncc.edu/content.php?pid=159011&sid=1345577

Weisman, D., & Zornado, J. (2012). *Professional writing for social work practice*. New York, NY: Springer.

Wood, L. (2014, January 6). The PhD's guide to a nonfaculty job search. *The Chronicle of Higher Education*, D4–D5. Retrieved from http://chronicle.com/article/The-PhDs-Guide-to-a/143715/

Young, J. (2009). *Designing interactive webinars: Principles and practice: A facilitator's perspective*. Retrieved from http://www.facilitate.com/support/facilitator-toolkit/docs/designing-interactive-webinars.pdf

# Writing for Publication: Assessment of a Course for Social Work Doctoral Students

DEENA MANDELL, HEND SHALAN, CAROL STALKER, and LEA CARAGATA

*Faculty of Social Work, Wilfrid Laurier University, Kitchener, Ontario, Canada*

*The authors describe a for-credit course for Social Work PhD students called Writing for Publication and report on a study evaluating its success in supporting students to develop and submit a paper for publication in a refereed journal. The literature-informed course design, taught in collaboration with the university's Writing Centre, includes didactic elements and a peer editing component. Seventeen of the 22 students who had taken the course completed an anonymous online survey asking whether they had submitted the paper and the outcome, whether the course had been helpful, in what ways, and in which other areas of the PhD program they were most helpful. The quantitative and qualitative data indicate that the course has been successful. A majority of students submitted an article to a peer-reviewed journal, and a majority found the course helpful in this regard as well as in other areas of the PhD program. Based on findings regarding the contributions of the course and student suggestions for improvement, we discuss considerations for strengthening the program in future.*

In September 2009, a mandatory new course called Writing for Publication was introduced into our Faculty of Social Work's doctoral curriculum. Its primary purpose was to support PhD students in preparing and submitting publishable papers. Our experiences with faculty hiring in recent years had shown us that applicants for positions in our faculty often had multiple publications in refereed journals, despite having just completed their PhD, or even having ABD status. We had also recognized that writing skills among all our students—MSW and PhD—generally were not at the level required for publication and were well aware that this was not unique to us. Having now offered the Writing for Publication course for five years, we set out to learn whether it has been fulfilling its mission and, if so, what modifications might be warranted.

In addition to positioning doctoral students advantageously in the academic market (Page-Adams, Cheng, Gogineni, & Shen, 1995), arguments in favor of publishing while in graduate programs include discovering "whether the life and work of a scholar are actually appealing" (McDougall & Stoilescu, 2010, p. 79), "enculturation" (Prior, 1995), and the related goal of "connecting with the research community" (McDougall & Stoilescu, 2010, p. 83). Although we acknowledge that pressure to publish at this stage may have some unwanted consequences (Crane & Pearson, 2011), there is growing evidence in the professional literature of efforts to systematically support doctoral student publication, and course syllabi are available online to do so in various disciplines.

## COURSE DESIGN INFORMED BY THE LITERATURE

Our course was developed by two faculty members with a particular interest in academic writing, one of whom had previously been involved in developing a set of writing workshops for MSW students in collaboration with the university's Writing Centre. The Writing for Publication doctoral option initially was offered as a single-term course. However, because most of the students required extensions lasting up to a full term longer in order to bring the paper to the expected standard, we subsequently spread the course out over two terms. The course syllabus was developed in consultation with the then-coordinator of the Writing Centre to draw on her expertise in academic writing and pedagogy. It was she who delivered content related to general academic writing principles, structure, and skills. Discipline-specific content was provided primarily by a social work instructor with guest participation by other faculty members. The mandatory course spans the fourth and fifth terms of the doctoral program, following completion of six other required courses.

Although establishing a community of practice has been inherent in the course design, the stated course objectives have been explicitly focused on the production of publishable academic manuscripts. These objectives are to

- develop an understanding of writing as a process, including identifying and developing an idea; writing an introduction and an abstract;

receiving, giving feedback, and rewriting; addressing fears, blocks, issues of voice; monitoring writing habits and other obstacles to writing in order to facilitate a productive process and experience;

- develop and submit a publishable manuscript;
- become aware of practical issues involved in getting a paper published;
- manage the interplay among creativity, disciplinary/academic discourse, and conventions and journal expectations;
- develop skills for line and structural editing, and use the skills to edit one's own and others' work;
- understand conventions related to different types of manuscripts, such as research reports (qualitative and quantitative), theoretical, practice based, etc.;
- offer, receive, and incorporate constructive criticism;
- acquire graduate-level technical writing skills appropriate for native and non-native English speakers;
- develop awareness of ethical issues relevant to scholarly publication.

The format for the course has included instructor presentation, a workshop process, and writing circles used to review ideas and writing with peers, to brainstorm ideas, and to give and receive constructive feedback (editorial and substantive) on writing. The configuration of these elements has been somewhat negotiable with each cohort, depending on their particular needs. The substantive content of the course has included the following elements:

- *Individual experience of writing: history, attitudes, and practical approaches*, which address students' current ideas, perceived personal and systemic strengths, barriers, and vulnerabilities. Students then are encouraged to reflect on the skills, knowledge, and resources they need in order to move forward with their writing project. Ethical issues potentially involved in publishing a paper also are discussed and students explore collectively what they will each need to consider.
- *Writing as a process* (taught by Writing Centre staff) focuses on identifying the purpose/contribution, audience, scope, and direction for the manuscript, as well as setting timelines. The need for an ongoing process of writing, reviewing, and editing/revising is explained. The purpose and advantages of a peer review process are delineated and the skills involved are introduced.
- *Purpose + Contribution → Audience.* At this point, the students begin applying the principles of academic writing to their respective projects. Individually, they begin reflecting on the gaps, problems, issues, and needs they want to address; who the audience is and what its priorities are (this includes identifying the appropriate target publication/funding body/conference); and formulation of a statement regarding the purpose,

contribution, and audience that will guide the student's thinking and writing. Students appear to find this early step far more challenging and far more significant to their progress than they had anticipated.

- *Elements of a successful paper* is a further module offered by Writing Centre staff. Elements include focus, authorial voice, structure (general and discipline specific), resources for guidelines on relevant conventions; writing a literature review; and key grammar issues, abstracts, and introductions.

- *Solo (vs.) collaborative writing* focuses on the advantages and potential disadvantages of each for academics in general, and more specifically for students and junior scholars. In the absence of firm rules regarding the management of shared authorship, the etiquette and ethics are discussed, particularly with regard to division of labour, order of authorship, control over input, and personal/professional boundaries.

- *Review process for journals* is focused on how the journals' review process works and associated timelines. "Dos and don'ts" regarding submission and communication with the journal also are covered. Dealing with feedback from the reviewers—both personally and professionally—is discussed and considerations relevant to revision and resubmission are explored. At this stage in the course, students are expected to have a short list of targeted journals that the group and the instructor then assist in narrowing down to the one that is most appropriate. These elements are consistent with Bender and Windsor's (2010) thoughts about "demystifying" the publication process for doctoral students in social work.

The peer group review component has been a central element of the Writing for Publication course. It begins very early in the course, as students give shape to the purpose and focus of their papers, and continues after the substantive content has been covered, while students work on developing their manuscripts. Writing and peer editing groups are becoming popular as a way of teaching students to offer and receive feedback on academic writing; they have been found to have some important advantages over feedback from the academic supervisor (Aitchison, 2009, 2010; Can & Walker, 2011; Cotterall, 2011). The actual skills developed are thought to derive not only from receiving critical feedback but also from learning to provide it (Aitcheson, 2009), so that the value of the group format goes beyond mere aggregation of input. Several authors also credit writing groups with broader social and intellectual development. As one authority notes, "Writing groups exemplify a pedagogy that realizes writing as a social practice because, in writing groups, writing is both produced through social interaction and is the outcome of social interaction" (Aitcheson, 2010, pp. 85–86). Furthermore, Can and Walker (2011) considered writing groups as "support systems to provide . . . safe environments for them to practice giving and receiving feedback" (p. 531).

In our groups, drafts or newly written sections of the student manuscripts were exchanged by e-mail among the group members, including the instructor, between meetings. When the group next met, everyone provided feedback to each person who had sent a manuscript out for peer review. The group met approximately every 2 to 3 weeks, but frequency varied, depending on the students' schedules and the progress they were able to make, given other demands on their time. (We sought balance between keeping the process moving and being mindful of the workload for doctoral students.) Other instructional strategies in the course included the use of relevant video material (in particular, a film called *Writing Across Borders* [Robertson, 2005], which addresses cross-cultural issues); provision of an extensive annotated bibliography in the syllabus; studying and deconstructing published writing examples; reflective exercises; and guest speakers, such as journal editors, a doctoral student who had published successfully and a university expert on intellectual property issues.

Students are given a passing grade after submitting a draft that the instructor deems ready for submission to a peer-reviewed journal, accompanied by the title of a selected journal and a written rationale for this choice. In some cases, the instructor may advise the student that further minor revisions are required, or would strengthen the manuscript, but administrative deadlines do not always allow for submission of another iteration of revision and review. In such cases, the student is assigned a passing grade and the student is advised to make the changes before submitting the manuscript.

Given the objectives and motivation behind the introduction of the course, our primary research question was: are students proceeding with submission of the articles written for the Writing for Publication course? Other questions were: Were the submissions ultimately accepted for publication? Which elements of the course were perceived to be useful, and in which areas of the PhD program were they most helpful? The research team consisted of three faculty members and one advanced doctoral candidate; two of the faculty members had been the instructors for the writing course, and one had been the administrator for the doctoral program from the time the course was first considered to the present.

The findings of our study are expected to be of general interest with respect to curriculum planning at both our own and other universities where a strong academic portfolio consisting of peer- reviewed publications is of increasing importance. Yet the task of writing for publication is one complicated by a student's own readiness, including having content of sufficient value to form the basis of a paper. A further interest is whether such a course of instruction proves beneficial, beyond the writing of this one required journal article, because this course is positioned just prior to students' undertaking their doctoral comprehensive paper and then their dissertation.

## METHOD

The data reported here were obtained through a purposeful survey of the 22 PhD students who had completed the mandatory doctoral-level course titled Writing for Publication. The sample population included both men and women, aged mid-20s to mid-50s, and encompassed students from abroad for whom English was not a first language. The proposal for the study was reviewed and approved by the university's Ethics Review Board. The survey was administered anonymously online through Survey Monkey, and no identifying information was sought or obtained. An e-mail was sent to all students who had been enrolled in the course from 2009 to 2013 with a letter of information explaining the study and inviting them to participate. The potential participants were advised that the questionnaire was voluntary, anonymous, and confidential and that it would take approximately 15 min to complete. Measures to protect anonymity were carefully explained.

The goals of the research (and hence the survey) were to determine the outcomes of the course with regard to publication and to obtain feedback from students regarding their experiences taking this course, particularly its helpfulness to them in progressing through the PhD program. To this end, the survey was comprised of 23 questions, of which 11 afforded respondents the opportunity to provide a short answer, clarification, or a comment on their experience. The remaining questions consisted of multiple-choice and Likert-type closed-end scales.

Given the course's orientation toward development and submission of a paper for publication to a peer-reviewed journal, most of the questions were oriented to inquiring about whether they were able to do this; the role of the course in improving their academic writing, difficulties encountered in achieving this course objective, and why these may have occurred. Data initially were analyzed via descriptive statistics utilizing SPSS, and all members of the team reviewed the results. Two composite scales were created and $t$ tests employed to test the significance of differences between subgroups of participants. Qualitative data were summarized and categorized thematically.

## FINDINGS

Seventeen of the 22 social work doctoral students who had been enrolled in Writing for Publication completed the survey, a response rate of 77.3%. (All but one had completed the course.) All agreed to the use of quotes from their written comments. Three of the 17 had successfully submitted a single sole-authored paper to a peer-reviewed journal *prior* to taking the course, leaving 14 (82.4%) who entered the course preparing to submit a sole-authored article for the first time.

## Submission of a Manuscript

In response to the question, "Did you submit the paper that you wrote for [this course] to a journal," 10 of the 17 students (58.8%) said they had submitted an article to a peer-reviewed journal, and the remaining seven (41.2%) said "not yet." The outcome of the 10 submissions (see Table 1) was that two were accepted, three were invited to revise and resubmit, and five were rejected.

When asked what they did next, all but one participant said that he or she had taken (or was in the process of taking) additional steps toward publication or making a formal conference presentation of the paper (see Table 2). Elsewhere in the survey, one student mentioned that s/he had not submitted a journal article but had successfully submitted a book chapter.[1]

In answer to the question "How long after the completion of the course did you submit the manuscripts?" six of the 10 (60%) said they submitted within 7 weeks, three (30%) within 2 to 3 months, and one took longer than 6 months to submit. (It's important to bear in mind that the first two cohorts

TABLE 1 What Was the Response From the Journal to Which You Originally Sent Your Article?

| Journal response | Frequency | % |
| --- | --- | --- |
| • Rejected | 5 | 29.4 |
| • Revise and submit | 3 | 17.6 |
| • Accepted with revision | 1 | 5.9 |
| • Accepted without revision | 1 | 5.9 |
| • Total | 10 | 58.8 |
| Missing | 7 | 41.2 |
| Total | 17 | 100.0 |

TABLE 2 What Did You Do Next?

| Action taken | Frequency | % |
| --- | --- | --- |
| • Did nothing further with it | 1 | 5.9 |
| • Currently working on revisions | 1 | 5.9 |
| • Revised and resubmitted to the same journal | 3 | 17.6 |
| • Revised and submitted to another journal | 3 | 17.6 |
| • Submitted to another journal | 1 | 5.9 |
| • Submitted to a conference or other similar forum | 1 | 5.9 |
| Total | 10 | 58.8 |
| Missing | 7 | 41.2 |
| Total | 17 | 100.0 |

---

[1]    We had unfortunately neglected to include submission of a chapter as an option for response to "What did you do next? [i.e. after hearing back from the journal]." The participant who submitted a chapter is not represented among the 10 who submitted to a peer-reviewed journal.

took the course in a single term but it was offered to subsequent cohorts across two terms. This may explain why some of the students indicated such a long time between the end of the course and submission.)

Those who took longer than 3 months to submit were asked, "What do you think contributed to the delay?" Only one of the two relevant students answered this, explaining that the article needed to be rewritten to "match the style of the journal." The question "What eventually enabled you to submit the paper?" was answered by six students and was more enlightening. Two students gave somewhat vague answers ("a rewrite" and "by the end of the course the paper was ready to submit"), but four credited review and feedback from the instructor with enabling completion, and two of those students also included feedback from peers.

At the time of survey completion, three[2] of the submitted articles had been accepted for publication in peer-reviewed journals and two of the papers had been presented at professional conferences. Three students indicated that they had subsequently submitted other papers to academic journals as well.

The students who indicated they had not resubmitted their manuscript to the original journal (or another) were asked to tell us why, and three responded; all referred to the discouragement of receiving a rejection, one recalling "harsh criticism regarding the ideas discussed" in the article.

We were, of course, interested to know what had gotten in the way of submission for the seven who had told us they had "not yet" submitted a paper. The responses to this question mainly pointed to lack of time and/or lack of priority. In addition, one student had not completed the course, and one had audited it (and thus, presumably, was not under pressure to complete a manuscript for the course credit). With a view to considering what changes might strengthen the course's helpfulness, we asked the nonsubmitters, "What do you think would need to happen in order for you to proceed with submitting the paper?" Some of the responses were consistent with the reasons for noncompletion: One student said that completing the course would have helped; two said they would need to get through their current stage of the program and find time to focus on the paper. Two others indicated that they could have used more help: One thought "more assistance from the instructor" was needed, and the other wrote, "writing labs, individual review and critique from professors who write in different journals/diverse writing genres, mentorship geared to the article, the journal and the individual student."

---

[2] At the time of writing this article, we have learned that an additional paper has been accepted, bringing the total to four of 10 articles accepted for publication to date. (The student who told one of the authors about this development had completed the survey.)

## Helpfulness of the Course for Article Submission

We wanted to know how helpful the students found each of the course's key elements as they were articulated in the course syllabus. For each element, students were asked to rate helpfulness on a 5-point Likert-type scale; the option of adding an element we had not listed also was offered, though none of the respondents chose to do so. The Cronbach's alphas for course helpfulness and course helpfulness for other academic writing were 0.97 and 0.76, respectively.

Figure 1 shows that the top five helpful elements were (a) writing and getting feedback from the instructor and revising; (b) developing the purpose/contribution, audience (intro), scope, and direction; (c) writing, getting feedback from peers, and revising; (d) overall structure; and (e) guidelines for reviewing/editing a draft. Fifteen of the 16 students (94.1%) who rated the element "Writing, getting feedback from the instructor, and revising" indicated it was helpful or somewhat helpful; one of the 16 indicated "uncertain" for this item, and no one said it was unhelpful. This is consistent with the student claims just reported that developing the paper toward submission readiness could have been helped by additional instructor input. It is also in keeping with the recommendations students offered about how we could improve the course, as we see next.

Eight students (53.3%) ranked "Writing, receiving feedback from instructors and revising" the most helpful, and no one ranked it least helpful. "Writing, receiving feedback from peers and revising," however, was rated

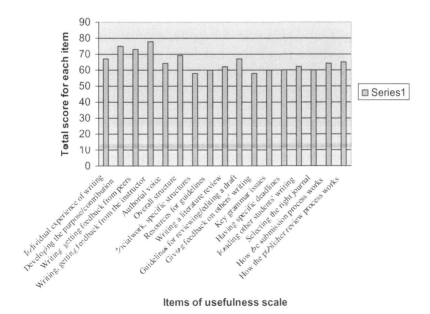

**Items of usefulness scale**

**FIGURE 1** Total scores of each item of the usefulness scale.

most helpful by three students but also least helpful by three. This led us to wonder whether students who submitted a paper might have seen the course as more helpful than students who did not. To answer this question, we developed a composite score for the students' ratings of the helpfulness of the course overall and assessed the normality of the scale.[3] An independent $t$ test was conducted to compare the Course Helpfulness scale for students who had submitted a paper to a journal and students who had not. No significant difference in scores for students who submitted a paper ($M = 65.8$, $SD = 18.95$) and students who did not was found ($M = 69.0$, $SD = 16.9$) at the specified .05 level, $t(13) = -.324$, $p = .751$.

No other course element received agreement from more than two respondents as either being most or least helpful, and several were not rated by anyone in this regard.

Twelve students responded to the question, "What do you think would have made this course more helpful to you?" Several of the comments were directed at the way the course is structured: One student said that advice on journal selection and "how the process works, i.e. the how to, not from just one professor, but as many genres as possible" would have made the course more useful. Two other students would have liked more individual feedback from the instructor as well, one of them specifically wanting the feedback to continue for a longer period. Another believed that co-authoring a paper with a faculty member would have been more helpful. One student would have liked "additional focus on structure and mechanics of writing," although the findings show that 12 out of 17 (71%) found the course element relating to overall structure to be helpful or somewhat helpful. Another student thought it would be more helpful "if students could start the course with a manuscript, instead of writing one during the course"; in fact, students now are encouraged to use a paper that has been written for a previous course as the starting point of the manuscript, and many are able to do this.

One particularly interesting comment challenged the viability of having students at widely disparate stages of writing ability and readiness working together, as this "makes it too difficult to move forward together and support one another usefully." We cannot know whether this particular student felt held back by others working more slowly or let down by those working at a quicker pace. Other responses focused on different ways in which the course could have been better; for example, one student wrote "having my own style and voice recognized"—perhaps a comment on the group editing process or possibly on perceived narrowness regarding acceptable writing styles. One who suggested longer duration of instructor involvement also recommended "social work specific structures." A student who likely took

---

[3]    The Course Helpfulness scale shows normal distribution as the Kolmogorov-Smirnov statistic shows nonsignificant result, with Sig. value equal to .200. This is also supported by a reasonably straight line in Normal Q-Q Plots.

the course when it was still a single-term offering said it would have been useful to know in advance that "it was going to take two terms." At that time, of course, even the instructors had no idea that it would take nearly everyone the better part of two terms to complete the paper to the required standard. One student said that completing a master's-level thesis[4] would have been helpful. Two students responded to this question by telling us how helpful the course had been for them. One of them said, "This course was extremely helpful and one of my favourites of the program" and the other wrote, "What stayed with me was the structure of a purpose statement and having the courage to develop your own voice in academic writing."

In response to the question, "What recommendations(s) do you have for strengthening the support offered to PhD students to submit work for publication?" a range of needs and perspectives were offered. Some of the responses to the previous question about what would have made the course more helpful were echoed here, such as individual faculty mentorship, involving as many faculty members as possible, more opportunities for joint publication, and continuing individual consultation with the instructor for a longer period, especially to deal with reviewer feedback from the journal. One student did not think ongoing assistance need necessarily come from the course instructor; options suggested (that already existed) were the student's advisor and staff of the Writing Centre. Another student suggested some form of ongoing facilitated writing group.

The final question of the survey encouraged students to add any comments/suggestions that they thought we should hear. We received eight responses. One of them, about the student's experience of the peer editing process, was somewhat troubling because of its implication that the process had been experienced as destructive in some way: "The group dynamics in the class were challenging. The instructor needs to maintain a very supportive culture and encourage constructive comments by all." Another student said, "I think the course slows us down because it takes a lot of us two terms to complete. I found that stressful with an already course-heavy PhD program." This was echoed by a student who said, "[Our] PhD program in SW has too many mandatory courses."

Three responses to the final question were highly positive about the students' experiences: One greatly appreciated the visit to class by a more senior doctoral student who had completed the Writing for Publication course and who has been particularly successful in getting papers accepted for publication. "Personal stories of successful students are very inspiring. . . ." The student who said s/he had not submitted an article to a peer-reviewed journal but had submitted a chapter to an edited volume was

---

[4]   Many students admitted to our PhD program have completed master's degree programs (in Social Work or related disciplines) in which there was no thesis requirement.

delighted to report that my chapter was accepted. I credit [this course] with easing the writing process for the chapter submission. . . . The skills I learned in [the course] helped me to be a better academic writer. I believe this course is an important one in the doctoral program.

A final student wrote, "I think this course is invaluable and I was lucky to take it!"

## Helpfulness of the Course for Other Academic Writing

As shown in Figure 2, in response to the statement about the primary objective of the course, participants were almost evenly divided about whether or not they would have been able to write a publishable article at that stage of the program without the course Although the course objectives did not explicitly target improvement of skills in other areas such as completing funding applications, writing the comprehensive proposal, comprehensive paper or the thesis proposal and dissertation themselves, we did ask the students whether they had found the course helpful in these areas. As also presented in Figure 2, the strongest agreement about helpfulness was in

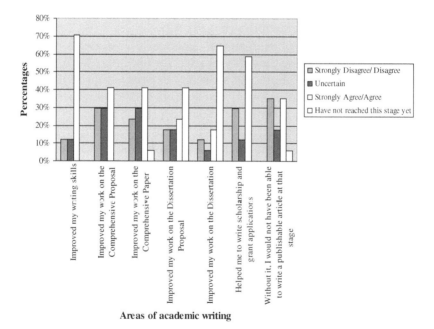

**FIGURE 2** Students' ratings of the helpfulness of the course for other areas of academic writing (*n* = 17). Only 16 participants rated the first and last items, "Improved my writing skills" and "Without it, I would not have been able to write a publishable article at that stage," respectively. The percentages for all items were calculated using 17 as the denominator for the purpose of comparison.

relation to scholarship and grant applications: Ten of the 17 respondents (58.8%) agreed or strongly agreed that the course had helped them to write these applications.

As we can also see in Figure 2, all participants had reached the comprehensive proposal stage; in all of these areas the course was considered by more students to be helpful than unhelpful. Three fourths of the respondents agreed or strongly agreed that the course had improved their writing skills overall, and nearly two thirds of them agreed or strongly agreed that it had been helpful with funding applications.

## DISCUSSION AND CONSIDERATIONS FOR THE FUTURE

Our findings indicate that a course offering doctoral students the experience of a supported writing project has been helpful to them in a number of ways: It has put producing a publication on their agenda earlier than might otherwise be the case and, for some, will have strengthened their profile as scholars by leading to publication by the time their dissertations are completed. The course also offers students skills applicable to writing grant and scholarship applications. For some, it was helpful in developing the comprehensive and thesis proposals, as well as the comprehensive paper and dissertation themselves. Unfortunately, due to the small sample size, we cannot say whether perceived unhelpfulness was an indicator of needing more help or simply not needing the help offered. The presence of three students among the participants who had submitted sole-authored manuscripts prior to taking the course speaks to this question. Nonetheless, within the small sample it is clear that individual needs and responses to the course often differed considerably.

The course element clearly identified as most helpful to the largest number was the reiteration of writing, receiving feedback from the instructor and revising. It is not surprising, therefore, that the primary way in which the respondents thought the course could be improved was to offer even more instructor feedback. Given the discouragement that some students expressed in the face of negative feedback received from journal reviewers—three to the point of abandoning the effort, at least temporarily—the idea of ongoing support makes a lot of sense. Even the most seasoned of scholars may know from painful personal experience that rejection, particularly when accompanied by harsh or dismissive reviewer comments, can make further work on a manuscript hard to contemplate. This prompts us to ask, Why not let the advisor assume this ongoing support? Depending on departmental and faculty culture, this approach might be a good way to see students through the stage of revision and resubmission, including the selection of an alternative journal, if appropriate. There are arguments in the literature both favoring and challenging this solution. Cotterall (2011) takes the position that faculty members should not be solely relied upon for adequate mentoring of students. In addition, some students' experience of the "asymmetrical power relations" with the members of their advisory committee may undermine their learning and their confidence as researchers (Cotterall, 2011, p. 423). On the other hand, Can and Walker (2011) found that 91% of their participants felt comfortable seeking feedback from committee members and 75% from their peers in the doctoral program (p. 520). Thus, having a dedicated faculty member (the course instructor) offering students writing support to the point of publication may in fact be the best approach. Although this would not satisfy the wish expressed by one participant for a wide range of faculty member involvement, it should be possible to invite more faculty members as guest speakers, or assemble a panel for a segment of the course, perhaps the one on journal selection.

The recommendation from a few of our participants that students be given more opportunity to publish jointly with faculty is inarguably ideal for some. Along with Can and Walker, we support this proposal where it is feasible; nevertheless, although it may bolster motivation and confidence (Can & Walker, 2011, p. 523) it may not enhance a graduate's curriculum vitae as greatly, or their capacity to write independently to the same extent as a sole authored publication.

Our participants' mixed responses regarding the helpfulness of the peer review process initially challenged our assumptions about the value of writing circles or peer group editing. The equal split in rating the experience of this course element's helpfulness, together with a number of the qualitative comments, was unexpected, and it led us to consider what might require modification in the way that the peer review component of the course presently is managed. There is enough evidence in the literature and in our own data regarding the value of writing groups that we cannot conclude the peer review process should be abandoned. One participant in our study commented that peer feedback—far from providing a "safe environment"— had an undermining effect; another wrote about the disparate needs and skills in the group being problematic. These comments led us to think more about the composition and dynamics of the peer review group and the role of the instructor as group facilitator. Aitchison (2010) prudently pointed out that facilitation should adapt to the needs of the participants, and certainly our students were at different stages of readiness for the course. Perhaps some of the additional individual help that several participants wished for could be offered at the front end of the course, allowing students then to proceed together as a group on more equal footing.

Participants' comments about the timing of the course present a conundrum. Specifically, given the usefulness of the course for writing funding applications, one student felt it should have been offered earlier, but this would be too soon for students to have done the coursework that would yield the material most rely upon to develop an article for publication.[5] It might serve all students' needs better if the course were separated into modules so that more immediately useful didactic elements (such as statement of purpose, audience, and scope) could be offered earlier in the program and other elements—especially peer review—could be introduced later. A peer review group for all interested doctoral students who had taken the writing course could be continued on a voluntary basis. If facilitation were needed, this might perhaps be another way to incorporate input from multiple faculty members. Those interested could be invited to volunteer for occasional facilitation.

In conclusion, a course in social work for doctoral students that combines didactic elements on academic writing and publication, instructor feedback, and peer group feedback appears to be helpful to most students. In addition to the desired outcome of submission of work for publication for more than half of them, most students strengthened their writing ability in other key areas of the doctoral program. Because instructor feedback was perceived to be valuable, continuing faculty support is warranted, and the peer review process, which received mixed evaluations, may benefit from modifications. With Crane and Pearson's (2011) lament in mind regarding the pressure to publish, we believe it is important to ensure that the writing course offers students as much support as possible in an environment conducive to their learning and their productivity.

## REFERENCES

Aitchison, C. (2009). Writing groups for doctoral education. *Studies in Higher Education, 34,* 905–916. doi:10.1080/03075070902785580

Aitchison, C. (2010). Learning together to publish: Writing group pedagogies for doctoral publishing. In C. Aitchison, B. Kamler, & A. Lee (Eds.), *Publishing pedagogies for the doctorate and beyond* (pp. 83–100). New York, NY: Routledge.

Bender, K., & Windsor, L. C. (2010). The four Ps of publishing: Demystifying publishing in peer-reviewed journals for social work doctoral students, *Journal of Teaching in Social Work, 30,* 147–158. doi:10.1080/08841231003697999

Can, G., & Walker, A. (2011). A model for doctoral students' perceptions and attitudes toward written feedback for academic writing. *Research in Higher Education, 52,* 508–536. doi:10.1007/s11162-010-9204-1

Cotterall, S. (2011). Doctoral students writing: Where's the pedagogy? *Teaching in Higher Education, 16,* 413–425. doi:10.1080/13562517.2011.560381

Crane, J., & Pearson, Z. (2011). Can we get a pub from this? Reflections on competition and the pressure to publish while in graduate school. *The Geographical Bulletin, 52,* 77–80.

---

[5]    Although grant-writing workshops are offered across the university, they do not address the kind of writing skills covered in the Writing for Publication course.

McDougall, D., & Stoilescu, D. (2010). Starting to publish academic research as a doctoral student. *International Journal of Doctoral Studies, 5*, 79–92.

Page-Adams, D., Cheng, L., Gogineni, A., & Shen, C. (1995). Establishing a group to encourage writing for publication among doctoral students. *Journal of Social Work Education, 31*, 102–107.

Prior, P. (1995). Tracing authoritative and internally persuasive discourses: A case study of response, revision, and disciplinary enculturation. *Research in the Teaching of English, 29*, 288–325.

Robertson, W. (Director) (2005). *Writing across borders* [Video]. Oregon State University Center for Writing and Learning and Writing Intensive Curriculum Program, University of Oregon, Corvallis, Oregon.

# Building Scholarly Writers: Student Perspectives on Peer Review in a Doctoral Writing Seminar

MARGARET ELLEN ADAMEK

*School of Social Work, Indiana University, Indianapolis, Indiana, USA*

*Peer review was used as a primary pedagogical tool in a scholarly writing course for social work doctoral students. To gauge student response to peer review and learning as a result of peer review, the instructor used narrative analysis to organize student comments into themes. Themes identified included initial trepidation, "no pain, no gain," and writing as relationship. Students transitioned from cautious reluctance about peer review to embracing it as a necessary part of the writing and publication process. As a profession that values collaboration, social work doctoral programs may benefit by encouraging peer support to enhance student writing and scholarly productivity.*

Quality scholarly publication is critical to the status of social work as a professional discipline. As early as 1915, Abraham Flexner asserted, "The evolution of social work toward . . . professional status can be measured by the quality of publication put forth in its name" (as cited in Sellers, Smith, Mathiesen, & Perry, 2006, p. 139). Despite the importance of scholarly publication to advancing knowledge of social work policy, practice, and education, studies of such publication in social work demonstrate unevenness in writing productivity. In essence, a relatively small group of social work scholars are very productive, whereas the larger group struggles to "do enough" (Fraser, 1994; Green, Baskind, Best, & Boyd, 1997).

These disparate patterns of productivity have been documented across disciplines (Furman & Kinn, 2011; Silvia, 2007). Citing a national survey of

40,000 faculty members conducted by the UCLA Higher Education Research Institute, Belcher (2009) reported that only about one fourth of faculty write regularly. Despite the widespread nature of writing struggles, some academics have a misperception that they are unique in their "writing dysfunction" (Belcher, 2009, p. 185). Apparently, the majority of academic writers resort to "binge writing" to accomplish necessary writing expectations (Furman & Kinn, 2011), an approach that has proven much less productive than ongoing scheduled writing (Boice, 1989).

Despite its importance to advancing the social work knowledge base and thus the professional status and contributions of the discipline, scholarly writing remains a silent struggle for many social work researchers. In their recommendations for promoting diversity in social work doctoral education, Schiele and Wilson (2001) called for doctoral programs to infuse content on scholarly writing in the curriculum. The centrality of publication to social work scholarship led one major Midwest school of social work to design and offer a doctoral course focused specifically on scholarly writing. A primary pedagogical tool used in the course was peer review.

Empirical studies conducted in the humanities have affirmed the value of peer review in the teaching and learning process (Ching, 2007; Flynn, 2008; Yang, 2011; Yuehchiu, 2007). Based on a historical analysis of peer review as a teaching tool, Ching (2007) pointed out that its use in composition classes dates back to the late 19th century. Peer review has been used successfully as well in a wide variety of courses including English as a Foreign Language (Yang, 2011), English composition (Ching, 2007; Chiu, Wang, & Wu, 2007; Yuehchiu, 2007), psychology (Cho, Schunn, & Charney, 2006; Covill, 2010), and educational leadership (Caffarella & Barnett, 2000). Doctoral students in educational leadership who participated in evaluating one "Scholarly Writing Project" in fact identified peer review as the most influential aspect of the course and of their learning about how to write for publication (Caffarella & Barnett, 2000). Examining peer review in an English writing course in Taiwan, Yang (2011) found that despite initial doubts about their peers' abilities, most students positively evaluated peer reviews of their writing. Students may also have reservations about their own reviewing ability (Chiu et al., 2007). Based on in-depth interviews with students in an English composition course, Yuehchiu (2007) concluded that multiple-draft revision is an important aspect of the peer review process and that students could benefit from training in peer response. In contrast to other studies, Covill (2010) found no difference in students' writing quality in an undergraduate psychology course under three conditions: formal peer review, self-review, and no review. Yuehchiu appropriately noted that there may be some cultural differences in students' acceptance of peer review.

Although peer review has been empirically supported as an effective pedagogical tool in several disciplines, its emergence in social work is more recent. A few social work educators have applied composition theory to teaching writing to social work students; however, the use of peer review was not emphasized (Dolejs & Grant, 2000; Waller, 2000). Nonetheless, one study conducted in a social work senior capstone course concluded that "peer mentoring techniques such as peer review and peer teaching appear to be a promising pedagogy that assists students in improving their writing skills and integrating their professional knowledge" (Badger, 2010, p. 16).

Combining their expertise in English and social work, Dolejs and Grant (2000) applied key concepts of composition theory in teaching writing to social work students. The concepts they identified were "writing to learn," "writing as process," and "writing as social act." Although the use of multiple drafts incorporates the concepts of "writing to learn" and "writing as process," peer review is aligned with the concept of "writing as social act." Writing to learn acknowledges that writing itself is a method of inquiry and thus a means of learning about a particular topic. Writing as process entails the understanding that good writing is fashioned over time and evolves in stages from a rough draft to a refined final product. Although the scholarly writing course described in this article used all of these three concepts from composition theory, this analysis focuses on peer review, and thus "writing as social act."

Further, other social work authors have reported that informal peer support through writing groups outside of the classroom is a helpful tool for promoting the scholarly productivity of both social work doctoral students (Page-Adams, Cheng, Gogineni, & Shen, 1995; Stratton, Upton-Davis, & Johnson, 2009) and faculty members (Bibus, Link, Rooney, Strom-Gottfried, & Sullivan, 1999). In a systematic review of factors facilitating dissertation completion specifically among social work doctoral students, Liechty, Liao, and Schull (2009) found that social support from both mentors and peers was critical to students' success. Although their analysis did not address peer review of writing specifically, Liechty et al. (2009) did point out (drawing from Vygotsky's sociocultural theory of learning) that "all learning occurs within the context of social interaction imbedded in a particular culture" (p. 487). Hence, peers, in essence, may become part of a "hidden curriculum" in doctoral programs (Liechty et al., 2009).

This inquiry focused on social work doctoral students' responses to using peer review in a course focused on scholarly writing. The project received an exemption from the university Institutional Review Board committee in February 2012 because data collected were part of the educational process, so informed consent was not required.

## METHODS

Since 2001, the author has taught a three-credit doctoral-level scholarly writing course every year. As of fall 2011, the course has been offered 12 times to a total of 81 doctoral students (58 female, 23 male). Those taking the course included 13 international and 13 racial minority students. The aim of the course is to equip students with the knowledge, skills, and motivation to be successful academic writers, including writing for publication. The primary assignment for the course is a progressive concept paper that students write in stages, beginning with a proposal. Early in the semester, students bring a one-page topic proposal to class to be circulated for review and comment. This ungraded assignment is the first opportunity in the course for "low-stakes" peer review (Elbow, 1997).

Prior to conducting in-class peer reviews, the instructor engages the students in a discussion of what constitutes constructive criticism. Students share their views about the type of feedback they most appreciate and that would likely be most helpful to them in the revision process. This discussion of the nature of constructive feedback establishes the expectations and guidelines students will follow in conducting a peer review. In addition, the instructor distributes several examples of reviewer guidelines from prominent scholarly journals. Likewise, students bring reviewer guidelines to class from a journal that may be a potential publication outlet for their paper.

Following Lamott's (1995) recommendations for writing, the instructor has the students produce a "down draft," or a first cut of their concept paper, with the notion of just getting something down. Students bring multiple copies of their down drafts to class for a peer review session. Students read and comment on each other's papers during class and take home one peer's paper to do a more thorough review. The following week, students submit the peer review they completed to the instructor and to the writer. Although students receive feedback and points on their written peer reviews, the down draft itself also is considered low-stakes writing (Elbow, 1997) and so is not graded. (Low-stakes writing includes drafts, concept mapping, outlining, and other forms of prewriting that are not subject to outcome evaluation.) Students revise their first drafts based on feedback from both their peers and the instructor. In a similar fashion, second drafts, or the "up draft" (Lamott, 1995) are brought to class about 4 weeks later for an in-class peer review. For a third time, therefore, students leave class with specific feedback from multiple peers. Each student conducts a second written peer review of another student's paper as a homework assignment. The final or "dental" draft (Lamott, 1995) is submitted to the instructor at the end of the semester for a grade. Lamott's use of the label "dental draft" implies the detailed editing of a final draft, cleaning up around all of the nooks and crannies. Thus, each student has at least three opportunities to receive input on his or her writing from peers, as well as from the instructor, as the papers progress from one draft to the next. In each case, the feedback is not anonymous, allowing students to follow up with their reviewers if they chose to do so. In some semesters, the instructor allowed class time for such "critical conversations," where student writers had a chance to discuss feedback with their peer reviewers. Given that this course is typically taken in the first semester of doctoral study, submitting the manuscript for publication is not a requirement. Nevertheless, a number of manuscripts that started out as concept papers in the course went on to be published, which is a desirable outcome (Burdge, 2007; Busch & Folaron, 2005; Deka, 2007; Lewis, 2007).

To examine student perceptions about peer review, the instructor conducted a careful review of students' written feedback about participating in this peer review process. First, students' written comments about peer review that were posted in online forums, in student self-evaluations of their writing progress, and in end-of-semester course evaluations were reviewed. Similar to the approach used by Cafferella and Barnett (2000), student comments were compiled, illustrating their reactions to peer review before, during, and after the peer review process. Next, content analysis was used to organize student feedback about peer review into themes. Representative student comments then were selected to illustrate each point of view. Ten themes were grouped under two broad categories: *challenges* of peer review and *benefits* of peer review. As might be expected, the challenges came mostly near the beginning of the peer review process, whereas the benefits typically were realized during and by the end of the course.

In considering the outcome, readers should remember that the student comments were not anonymous. The instructor's enthusiasm for peer review as a teaching tool in the scholarly writing course therefore could have influenced students' feedback. Moreover, because the students' comments noted in this paper were drawn from a convenience sample of social work doctoral students from one university, they cannot be considered representative of the views of all doctoral students regarding peer review as a learning tool.

# FINDINGS

## Challenges

### INITIAL TREPIDATION

At the outset of the course, students seemed to have low expectations of peer review. Comments included "opening myself up to others seemed threatening" and "feeling uncomfortable receiving feedback from my peers." Feelings of stress, anxiety, apprehension, and vulnerability were common early on in the course. Some students were concerned about their peers' ability to give constructive feedback and expressed reluctance about the prospect of giving negative feedback to their peers. Of interest, students were fine with the instructor reading their work, because that was expected, but considered the idea of having their classmates read their papers "an extra level of pressure."

## "No Pain, No Gain"

Several students acknowledged that, despite the initial affective response that came with receiving constructive criticism of their writing, their papers did improve as a result. As one student stated, "Honest feedback, although sometimes painful, has lead not only to refinements, but to gains." Although the first reading of peer feedback may have been difficult for some students to accept, they came to see the value of having multiple reviewers. "Getting past my initial twinge reaction, I can now listen to what is being said." Another opined, "The peer review process, although initially painful, provided a preview of the probable reaction from other reviewers. Although the feedback proved valuable in reworking the paper, the experience was not for the weak-hearted." In time, however, students learned to "get past the emotional impact of the review."

Students noted that their initial reaction to constructive feedback often was negative, even when both positive and negative feedback were given. As one student shared, "I noticed how sensitive we are to anything that seems negative, zeroing in on the one or two [critical] comments while glossing over the encouragement and support." Appreciation for peer comments improved over time. "Each time I received feedback it became a little easier, but I still struggle with remembering that the point is to help improve my writing so my message can be clearly delivered."

## Transformation in Thinking

After multiple experiences with peer review during the course, student reactions transitioned from initial trepidation to becoming appreciative, and even enthusiastic. Several student comments reflected their change of heart about receiving feedback on their writing from their peers. One observed, "A willingness to participate in peer review has improved as experience has underscored the importance of the process." Students increasingly saw the supportive nature of critical comments. As one stated, "Each [peer review] experience will improve my ability to see criticism as a kindness extended by a peer, not to be taken as some type of personal attack." Students' affective response to peer review changed as well: "My comfort level and confidence in allowing others to review/critique my writing increased." Judging by students' comments, it seems that multiple opportunities for peer feedback were integral to bringing about the transformation. One sensitively stated, "So much feedback has caused a de-sensitization to having others read my writing which was the source of much of my anxiety," whereas another remarked that "this kind of constant peer review is taking away a lot of the 'sting' or 'vulnerability' experienced in the past when putting my writing on the chopping block." One doctoral student summed it up well: "The more I experience the process, the more natural it seems."

## BENEFITS

Student comments about peer review, especially toward the end of the course, revealed benefits of the process that students generally did not anticipate at the outset. These perceived benefits were grouped into seven subthemes: appreciation/mutual support, gaining insight about one's own writing, producing a better written product, broadening one's perspective, heightened sensitivity to one's readers, seeing writing as a relationship, and excitement about making an impact in the future.

### Appreciation/Mutual Support

Despite their initial expectations, students came to appreciate feedback from peers and to conceptualize it as a form of mutual support. As one student shared, "I did not expect to feel the mutual support ... given through encouragement and feedback that others were willing to give." Some students were pleasantly surprised by the helpfulness of their peers' comments: "Going back to the comments at a later time, I found them very helpful." Students began to realize that they did not have to fear their peers' input: "The reviewer's extensive feedback was supportive and some recommendations matched the instructor's [advice]." They came to appreciate the opportunity "to correct some of the beginner's mistakes without consequences."

### Gaining Insight About One's Own Writing

A second benefit identified from students' comments was the opportunity to gain insight about one's own writing style. One student acknowledged that "the feedback could be used as a gauge in terms of how well I expressed my thoughts." Based on input from peers, students came to recognize specific shortcomings in their own writing. For example, one student acknowledged that "(reviewer) questions challenged me to look at sources or concepts more closely and to decide if clarification or support were needed." Another noted that peer review "helps me to be more mindful of clarity." "Through the peer review process, I have learned that my writing has some vocabulary, construction, and logical flow-related issues that make assimilation of my ideas difficult for the reader." In addition, students began to positively appreciate the contributions they were capable of making through their writing.

Both aspects of the peer review process—receiving feedback and providing feedback—were noted by students as avenues for strengthening their writing: "Having to edit others' work has increased my ability to write in a concise manner." Another shared, "Having my peers read and review my writing, as well as having the opportunity to read the work of others, has helped me to identify strengths and areas for improvement in my own writing. . . . I am better able to recognize [my] flaws and mistakes."

## Producing a Better Product

As students continued to rework and revise their concept papers, based on input from peers, they came to realize how much the feedback they received helped them to produce a better written product. One student noted, "I have found that the input they gave can be invaluable in editing my manuscript and further polishing a finished product." Peer feedback was credited by students for "achieving greater clarity" in their writing and "strengthening" and "improving the final outcome" of their papers. Along with this process, the class discussed the statement, "All writing is revision," and thereby came to view revision not as a remedial task to shore up weak writing but as a necessary and inevitable step for producing clear and powerful prose. Students acknowledged developing a deeper respect for revision: "I knew [revision] was important, but I generally thought I was meticulous enough . . . to not have to go back and spend much time with revision. I now have a deep respect for peer review and the power of revision." Given the opportunity to incorporate input, from both peers and the instructor, on multiple drafts, students generally felt more confident about the quality of their final papers. The instructor as well noticed marked (and sometimes remarkable) improvements in students' writing from the first to the final draft.

## Broadening One's Perspective

Peer review also offered the doctoral students an opportunity to broaden their perspective about their own topics. Many acknowledged that the peer critique process helped them "to gain additional perspectives" and "offer a fresh viewpoint." Some realized that their own writing could be strengthened when it incorporated other perspectives they had not anticipated. As one student noted, "There were several ideas presented by my classmates that I had not previously considered. Their input will help me facilitate a critical review of my proposal."

## Heightened Sensitivity to Readers

An additional benefit of peer review was a heightened sensitivity to readers. Peer review was acknowledged as "a way to test the waters and preview what the reaction might be from a larger audience." Questions on their drafts challenged students to consider that "the reader might not understand" their underlying premise or subject matter. One student wrote, "I think it is very natural for writers to assume that they have clearly stated their point when in fact the reader may be confused about their stance." Students became more mindful when writing for an audience. As one stated, "Knowing what the reader is looking for or expecting is a great advantage to writing in a more impactful way." As another student noted, "I want to write for my reader. I want it to be well-understood and to inform—perhaps even enlighten."

## Writing as Relationship

Although the tendency of academic writers is to view writing as a solitary process, via peer review, students came to see that "professional writing skills are developed through interaction with others." Although acknowledging that "scholarly writing is technical," students noted that "it also requires an integration of personal and creative thoughts." They acknowledged a change in their perception about writing from an activity that is "isolated, technical, and personally detached" to involving "shared learning, creativity, and personal connections." Although they all were writing solo-authored papers, students came to conceptualize their peers as partners in developing their writing skills. In contrast to their initial reluctance to receiving peer feedback, students came to see fellow students as writing allies: "I am beginning to feel that my classmates and I are on the same journey and that we are trying to encourage one another and help each one of us to be successful." This perception and feeling is a tribute to what group workers would term the power of mutual aid.

## Excitement for Making an Impact

As they experienced the benefits of peer review, students became increasingly eager to seek out peer support through writing groups and accountability partners, beyond the 15-week semester. They often noted the value of peer review for their future scholarly efforts, including the completion of their degree: "The shift in my relationship with peer review will serve me well as the PhD process continues." Students' growing appreciation for the value of peer review sparked hopeful attitudes about their future scholarly endeavors: "Instead of being afraid to disappoint someone, or looking unintelligent, I hope to gain feedback on my writing so I can one day become published." Similarly, another wrote, "Developing comfort with peer review and constructive criticism will also prepare me for my future publishing efforts." Further, one student put it this way: "My competition is not with my classmates. My competition is with me—to become a better writer and to write ideas that someone wants to read and that can have a positive impact on someone's life." In considering the larger context of scholarly writing, one student commented,

> We represent not only ourselves in our work, but our profession as a
> whole. I have learned that we need to be careful and conscientious in

how we present our ideas, not only in word choice and flow, but in structure. I am inspired to imagine my work as exemplary of our social work profession, creating a positive impact in people's lives.

## DISCUSSION

A one-semester course on scholarly writing offered to social work doctoral students saw most students transformed from reluctant participants to enthusiasts for peer review. Despite some resistance to the initial acceptance of the peer review process, the benefits of peer review, as illustrated by students' own comments, proved to be multiple and varied. As indicated by students' own reflections, the advantages of peer review in terms of promoting clarity and critical thinking in students' written products appeared to outweigh the challenges of incorporating peer review into the course. In the process of revising their writing, students obtain feedback from more than one perspective; the instructor's perspective is not considered as the only valid one. As Bender and Windsor (2010) acknowledged, social work doctoral students clearly offer new perspectives, energy, and enthusiasm to the scholarly writing process.

The value of peer review should be further investigated and confirmed through research at other universities. Although the use of students' own comments about peer review was one of the strengths of this study, further exploration is needed to examine the impact of peer review on the quality of social work students' writing and scholarly productivity. In addition, this study was not able to document whether the use of peer review in a class setting led to the pursuit of peer review to support writing beyond the course itself. Although several students offered both verbal and written comments about their hopes to continue to actively participate in peer review, their later actions in this regard were not tracked.

## CONCLUSION

Peer review is highly recommended as a strategy to enhance doctoral students' scholarly writing. Based on comments from participants, this inquiry leads us to believe that peer review may be an effective mechanism for supporting student writing. Students here transitioned from fearing the feedback of their classmates to viewing their peers as allies in the writing process. They learned to push past the initial twinge reaction to input, perceived as critical, to welcome and even seek out the feedback of peers. As students accepted that peer review was a critical avenue for clarifying and strengthening their writing, they became more sensitive to writing for an audience, an approach that is integral to successful scholarship (Hyland, 2001). In this sense we incorporated principles touted by Gopen (2004) about writing from the readers' perspective. Instead of being a lonely endeavor or "silent struggle," it was shown that scholarly writing could become a shared effort involving mutual aid and collegial support. Moreover, through interaction with peers, the challenges of writing, rather than being perceived as unique, were normalized.

As a profession that values collaboration, social work can encourage peer support of writing—both in classroom exercises and on manuscripts for publication. In their evaluation of the helpfulness of peer comments, Cho et al. (2006) noted that peer review promotes "an active writing community" among students (p. 280). Peer support and collaboration may thus promote the dissemination of scholarly contributions of a broader range of social work scholars, beyond the usual small set of prolific writers. The profession will benefit when a wider range of perspectives is voiced through published work. In sum, peer support of scholarly writing in doctoral programs may serve to advance and enrich the social work knowledge base, thus strengthening the stature and contributions of the profession.

## REFERENCES

Badger, K. (2010). Peer teaching and review: A model for writing development and knowledge synthesis. *Social Work Education, 29*, 6–17. doi:10.1080/02615470902810850

Belcher, W. L. (2009). Reflections on ten years of teaching writing for publication to graduate students and junior faculty. *Journal of Scholarly Publishing, 40*, 184–200. doi:10.3138/jsp.40.2.184

Bender, K., & Windsor, L. C. (2010). The four *P*s of publishing: Demystifying publishing in peer-reviewed journals for social work doctoral students. *Journal of Teaching in Social Work, 30*, 147–158. doi:10.1080/08841231003697999

Bibus, A., Link, R., Rooney, R., Strom-Gottfried, K., & Sullivan, M. (1999). The writer's group. *Families in Society: The Journal of Contemporary Social Services, 80*, 531–534. doi:10.1606/1044-3894.1483

Boice, R. (1989). Procrastination, busyness, and bingeing. *Behaviour Research and Therapy, 27*, 605–611. doi:10.1016/0005-7967(89)90144-7

Burdge, B. (2007). Bending gender, ending gender: Theoretical foundations for social work practice with the transgender community. *Social Work, 52*, 243–250. doi:10.1093/sw/52.3.243

Busch, M., & Folaron, G. (2005). Accessibility and clarity of state child welfare mission statements. *Child Welfare, 84*, 415–430.

Caffarella, R. S., & Barnett, B. G. (2000). Teaching doctoral students to become scholarly writers: The importance of giving and receiving critiques. *Studies in Higher Education, 25*, 39–52. doi:10.1080/030750700116000

Ching, K. L. (2007). Peer response in the composition classroom: An alternative genealogy. *Rhetoric Review, 26*, 303–319. doi:10.1080/07350190701419863

Chiu, C., Wang, C., & Wu, W. (2007). Examining the effects of two combined peer and teacher feedback models on college students' writing quality. *International Journal of the Humanities*, *5*(5), 43–50.

Cho, K., Schunn, C. D., & Charney, D. (2006). Commenting on writing: Typology and perceived helpfulness of comments from novice peer reviewers and subject matter experts. *Written Communication*, *23*, 260–294. doi:10.1177/0741088306289261

Covill, A. E. (2010). Comparing peer review and self-review as ways to improve college students' writing. *Journal of Literacy Research*, *42*, 199–226. doi:10.1080/10862961003796207

Deka, A. (2007). Conceptualizing gender equity in the Indian health care system. *Perspectives on Social Work*, *6*, 21–24.

Dolejs, A., & Grant, D. (2000). Deep breaths on paper: Teaching writing in the social work classroom. *Journal of Teaching in Social Work*, *20*(3–4), 19–40. doi:10.1300/J067v20n03_04

Elbow, P. (1997). High stakes and low stakes in assigning and responding to writing. In M. D. Sorcinelli & P. Elbow (Eds.), *Writing to learn: Strategies for assigning and responding to writing across the disciplines* (pp. 5–13). San Francisco, CA: Jossey-Bass.

Flynn, D. (2008). Using peer-review effectively in large, diverse classes. *International Journal of the Humanities*, *5*(11), 65–81.

Fraser, M. (1994). Scholarship and research in social work: Emerging challenges. *Journal of Social Work Education*, *30*, 252–266.

Furman, R., & Kinn, J. T. (2011). *Practical tips for publishing scholarly articles: Writing and publishing in the helping professions* (2nd ed.). Chicago, IL: Lyceum.

Gopen, G. (2004). *Expectations: Teaching writing from the reader's expectations.* New York, NY: Pearson/Longman.

Green, R. G., Baskind, F. R., Best, A. M., & Boyd, A. S. (1997). Getting beyond the productivity gap: Assessing variation in social work scholarship. *Journal of Social Work Education*, *33*, 541–553.

Hyland, K. (2001). Bringing in the reader: Addressee features in academic articles. *Written Communication*, *18*, 549–574. doi:10.1177/0741088301018004005

Lamott, A. (1995). *Bird by bird: Some instructions on writing and life.* New York, NY: Doubleday.

Lewis, L. (2007). No-harm contracts: A review of what we know. *Suicide & Life-Threatening Behavior*, *37*, 50–57. doi:10.1521/suli.2007.37.1.50

Liechty, J. M., Liao, M., & Schull, C. P. (2009). Facilitating dissertation completion and success among doctoral students in social work. *Journal of Social Work Education*, *45*, 481–497. doi:10.5175/JSWE.2009.200800091

Page-Adams, D., Cheng, L., Gogineni, A., & Shen, C. (1995). Establishing a group to encourage writing for publication among doctoral students. *Journal of Social Work Education*, *31*, 402–407.

Schiele, J. H., & Wilson, R. G. (2001). Issues and guidelines for promoting diversity in doctoral social work education. *Arete*, *25*, 53–66.

Sellers, S. L., Smith, T., Mathiesen, S. G., & Perry, R. (2006). Perceptions of professional social work journals: Findings from a national survey. *Journal of Social Work Education*, *42*, 139–160. doi:10.5175/JSWE.2006.200303095

Silvia, P. (2007). *How to write a lot: A practical guide to productive academic writing.* Washington, DC: American Psychological Association.

Stratton, K., Upton-Davis, K., & Johnson, C. (2009). A writer's circle: Spiraling into print. *Families in Society: The Journal of Contemporary Social Services, 90,* 1–4. doi:10.1606/1945-1350.3864

Waller, M. (2000). Addressing student writing problems: Applying composition theory to social work education. *Journal of Baccalaureate Social Work, 5,* 161–166.

Yang, S. (2011). Exploring the effectiveness of using peer evaluation and teacher feedback in college students' writing. *Asia-Pacific Education Researcher, 20,* 144–150.

Yuehchiu, F. (2007). The effects of peer reviews in EFL college composition classes: From learners' perspectives. *International Journal of the Humanities, 5,* 137–142.

# CONCLUSION

# Doctoral Education in Social Work: An Essay Review

*College of Social Work, Florida State University, Tallahassee, Florida, USA*

Jeanne W. Anastas. (2012). *Doctoral Education in Social Work*. New York, NY: Oxford University Press (271 pp., $36.00, paperback, ISBN# 978-0-19-537806-1).

Quality doctoral education is critical to the intellectual health and growth of the evidence-based foundations of the social work profession. Most social work doctorates are research focused but, unlike the MSW and BSW practice degrees, lack formal accreditation. Thus, quality control remains the sole prerogative of individual programs and their host universities. Although the Group for the Advancement of Doctoral Education in Social Work (GADE) sponsors an annual meeting of doctoral program directors and publishes some important documents on doctoral education, it has no regulatory authority and membership in GADE is voluntary. Meanwhile, the Council on Social Work Education, the group with actual monitoring influence and accreditation authority in social work education, focuses largely on BSW and MSW programs. Moreover, in contrast to the humanities, social work programs graduate fewer PhDs than there are available faculty positions. Clearly doctoral education in American social work has significant lacunae.

In 2007, Dr. Anastas, past president of the National Association of Social Workers and GADE, undertook a comprehensive survey of doctoral social work students enrolled that year. Her online cross-sectional study collected data about the doctoral student experience in the United States and Canada. Survey questions inquired about student demographics and professional backgrounds; admissions and enrollment variables; doctoral programs and financial support; and some proximate outcomes such as time in a program, student satisfaction, and career goals. Of the 801 anonymous responses received, incomplete surveys were common due to the survey's length. Still, a very rich pool of information was collected from the mix of quantitative and qualitative questions.

The book is organized in accordance with the survey's major themes. Following two introductory chapters, describing the need for and design of this study, and the landscape of doctoral education, Chapter 3 summarizes the data on *admissions, recruitment, and enrollment*; Chapter 4 discusses *paying for doctoral education*; Chapter 5 describes the *students' experiences and satisfaction with doctoral study;* and Chapter 6 draws on "student experience" data regarding the *dissertation research experience, academic advising, and preliminary examinations.* Chapter 7 subsequently summarizes the data on *postdoctoral career preparation* including teaching, publishing, and finding academic and nonacademic positions. Some proximal outcomes of doctoral education are then reviewed in Chapter 8, including a set of interesting regression analyses. The final chapter draws conclusions, suggests implications, and outlines some future challenges.

With its literature review, comprehensive online survey, data collection, and data analysis, this book is a real accomplishment. I earnestly hope that someone—Dr. Anastas, GADE, the Council on Social Work Education, the Society for Social Work and Research, or even NASW—commits to keeping this resource alive, periodically replicating the original study so that a one-time cross-sectional survey evolves into a longitudinal database. The few published studies on this topic are quite limited (e.g., Artelt & Thyer, 2009; Crowe & Kindelsperger, 1975; Thyer & Barker, 2003). (I wish, parenthetically, that the actual survey had been published as an appendix in the book—though Anastas will provide a copy upon request.) A replication might expand the sample to include recent graduates, for example, allowing for an analysis of benchmarks like graduation, publication, and employment. Such a replication also could focus productively on curriculum (a regrettable omission in the Anastas study), as it forms the core of all doctoral education. Doctoral programs' use of, and individual respondents' scores on, the Graduate Record Exam (GRE) are missing. Because GRE scores are widely used yet controversial (Donahue & Thyer, 1993; Thyer & Barker, 2003) as an admission criterion, an examination of this variable's descriptive features and correlates would have enhanced the discussion. Of course, the results might have been embarrassing, as social work graduate students consistently rank among the lowest national scorers on the GRE (Stoesz, Karger, & Carrilio, 2010). Yet embarrassing data are still useful data.

The survey's findings are amply illustrated with quotes from the respondents, providing a potentially rich lode of qualitative information. However, the data seem to have been indifferently mined. Because Anastas did not include her methodology for analyzing the narrative comments, the remarks are of unknown credibility. This is a regrettably common practice in qualitative research, and the possibility therefore remains that the author selected comments that inadvertently reflect personal biases, reinforcing the widespread (but incorrect) perception that qualitative methods are inherently less empirical. Although this may not be true of this book, Anastas's championing of qualitative research (Anastas, 2012) makes her lack of narrative analysis here regrettable.

The author's survey is a sterling example of a purely empirical yet highly valuable descriptive study. Nevertheless, this descriptive study lacks an overall organizing conceptual framework. No reference is made to pedagogical theory or to hypotheses derived from theory and prospectively tested, speculation about student decision making, or any psychosocial or environment predictors of program completion. Our field has long benefited from theory-free research of this type, just as it has profited from theoretically driven investigations. Both forms of scientific inquiry have their value, as it has been noted elsewhere (Thyer, 2001), and the field should now cease its misguided elevation of trivial theoretical studies at the expense of theory-free investigations.

I believe that both doctoral faculty and students will find this book absorbing reading, inasmuch as it is presently the largest study of its type in our field and a substantial improvement on earlier works (e.g., Holland & Frost, 1987; Lowenberg, 1972; Regensburg, 1966; Rosen & Stretch, 1982). The findings are rarely surprising, and they corroborate commonly held views, but to add substantive data to these views is an exceptionally useful undertaking and one liable to be highly cited in years to come. Anastas possesses the gift of integrating her new empirical data with extent prior studies, which makes her findings even more useful by placing them in a larger historical and empirical context.

# REFERENCES

Anastas, J. (2012). From scientism to science: How contemporary epistemology can inform practice research. *Clinical Social Work Journal, 40*, 157–165. doi:10.1007/s10615-012-0388-z

Artelt, T., & Thyer, B. A. (2009). A comparison of the academic performance of experienced versus inexperienced MSWs earning the social work doctorate: An exploratory study. *Korean Journal of Social Welfare Research, 20*, 1–32.

Crowe, R. T., & Kindelsperger, K. W. (1975). The PhD or the DSW? *Journal of Education for Social Work, 11*(3), 38–43. doi:10.1080/00220612.1975.10778699

Donahue, B., & Thyer, B. A. (1993). Should the GRE be used as an admissions requirement by schools of social work? *Journal of Teaching in Social Work, 6*(2), 33–40. doi:10.1300/J067v06n02_04

Holland, T. P., & Frost, A. K. (1987). *Doctoral education in social work: Trends and issues* (Social Work Education Monograph Series). Austin: University of Texas at Austin.

Lowenberg, F. M. (1972). *Doctoral education in schools of social work.* New York, NY: Council on Social Work Education.

Regensburg, J. (1966). *Some educational patterns in doctoral programs in schools of social work.* New York, NY: Council on Social Work Education.

Rosen, A., & Stretch, J. (Eds.). (1982). *Doctoral education in social work: Issues, perspectives, and evaluation.* St. Louis, MO: Group for the Advancement of Doctoral Education in Social Work.

Stoesz, D., Karger, H. J., & Carrilio, T. (2010). *A dream deferred: How social work education lost its way and what can be done.* New Brunswick, NJ: Aldine Transaction

Thyer, B. A. (2001). What is the role of theory in research on social work practice? *Journal of Social Work Education, 37,* 9–25.

Thyer, B. A., & Barker, K. L. (2003). A bibliography of doctoral education in social work. In B. A. Thyer & T. G. Arnold (Eds.), *A program guide to doctoral study in social work* (pp. 168–175). Alexandria, VA: CSWE. [A copy of this bibliography covering (1952–2002) is available from the author.]

# Index

INDEX